Medical Statistics at a Glance

Medical Statistics at a Glance

AVIVA PETRIE

Senior Lecturer in Statistics
Biostatistics Unit
Eastman Dental Institute for Oral Health Care Sciences
University College London
256 Grays Inn Road
London WC1X 8LD *and*
Honorary Lecturer in Medical Statistics
Medical Statistics Unit
London School of Hygiene and Tropical Medicine
Keppel Street
London WC1E 7HT

CAROLINE SABIN

Senior Lecturer in Medical Statistics and Epidemiology
Department of Primary Care and Population Sciences
The Royal Free and University College Medical School
Royal Free Campus
Rowland Hill Street
London NW3 2PF

Blackwell
Science

© 2000 by Blackwell Science Ltd
a Blackwell Publishing company
Blackwell Science, Inc., 350 Main Street, Malden, Massachusetts 02148-5018, USA
Blackwell Publishing Ltd, 9600 Garsington Road, Oxford OX4 2DQ, UK
Blackwell Science Asia Pty Ltd, 550 Swanston Street, Carlton South, Victoria 3053, Australia
Blackwell Wissenschafts Verlag, Kurfürstendamm 57, 10707 Berlin, Germany

First published 2000
Reprinted 2001, 2001, 2002, 2003

Library of Congress Cataloging-in-Publication Data

Petrie, Aviva.
  Medical statistics at a glance / Aviva Petrie, Caroline Sabin.
     p.   cm.
  Includes index.
  ISBN 0-632-05075-6
  1. Medical statistics.   2. Medicine — Statistical methods.
  I. Sabin, Caroline.   II. Title.   ·
R853.S7 P476   2000
610´.727—dc21   99-045806

ISBN 0-632-05075-6

A catalogue record for this title is available from the British Library

Set by SNP Best-set Typesetter Ltd., Hong Kong
Printed and bound in the UK at
TJ International Ltd, Padstow

For further information on Blackwell Publishing, visit our website:
http://www.blackwellpublishing.com

Contents

Preface

Medical Statistics at a Glance is directed at undergraduate medical students, medical researchers, postgraduates in the biomedical disciplines and at pharmaceutical industry personnel. All of these individuals will, at some time in their professional lives, be faced with quantitative results (their own or those of others) that will need to be critically evaluated and interpreted, and some, of course, will have to pass that dreaded statistics exam! A proper understanding of statistical concepts and methodology is invaluable for these needs. Much as we should like to fire the reader with an enthusiasm for the subject of statistics, we are pragmatic. Our aim is to provide the student and the researcher, as well as the clinician encountering statistical concepts in the medical literature, with a book that is sound, easy to read, comprehensive, relevant, and of useful practical application.

We believe *Medical Statistics at a Glance* will be particularly helpful as a adjunct to statistics lectures and as a reference guide. In addition, the reader can assess his/her progress in self-directed learning by attempting the exercises on our Web site (www.medstatsaag.com), which can be accessed from the Internet. This Web site also contains a full set of references (some of which are linked directly to Medline) to supplement the references quoted in the text and provide useful background information for the examples. For those readers who wish to gain a greater insight into particular areas of medical statistics, we can recommend the following books:

Altman, D.G. (1991) *Practical Statistics for Medical Research.* Chapman and Hall, London.
Armitage, P., Berry, G. (1994) *Statistical Methods in Medical Research*, 3rd edn. Blackwell Scientific Publications, Oxford.
Pocock, S.J. (1983) *Clinical Trials: A Practical Approach.* Wiley, Chichester.

In line with other books in the *At a Glance* series, we lead the reader through a number of self-contained, two- and three-page topics, each covering a different aspect of medical statistics. We have learned from our own teaching experiences, and have taken account of the difficulties that our students have encountered when studying medical statistics. For this reason, we have chosen to limit the theoretical content of the book to a level that is sufficient for understanding the procedures involved, yet which does not overshadow the practicalities of their execution.

Medical statistics is a wide-ranging subject covering a large number of topics. We have provided a basic introduction to the underlying concepts of medical statistics and a guide to the most commonly used statistical procedures. Epidemiology is closely allied to medical statistics. Hence some of the main issues in epidemiology, relating to study design and interpretation, are discussed. Also included are topics that the reader may find useful only occasionally, but which are, nevertheless, fundamental to many areas of medical research; for example, evidence-based medicine, systematic reviews and meta-analysis, time series, survival analysis and Bayesian methods. We have explained the principles underlying these topics so that the reader will be able to understand and interpret the results from them when they are presented in the literature. More detailed discussions may be obtained from the references listed on our Web site.

There is extensive cross-referencing throughout the text to help the reader link the various procedures. The Glossary of terms (Appendix D) provides readily accessible explanations of commonly used terminology. A basic set of statistical tables is contained in Appendix A. Neave, H.R. (1981) *Elementary Statistical Tables* Routledge, and *Geigy Scientific Tables* Vol. 2, 8th edn (1990) Ciba-Geigy Ltd., amongst others, provide fuller versions if the reader requires more precise results for hand calculations.

We know that one of the greatest difficulties facing non-statisticians is choosing the appropriate technique. We have therefore produced two flow-charts which can be used both to aid the decision as to what method to use in a given situation and to locate a particular technique in the book easily. They are displayed prominently on the inside cover for easy access.

Every topic describing a statistical technique is accompanied by an example illustrating its use. We have generally obtained the data for these examples from collaborative studies in which we or colleagues have been involved; in some instances, we have used real data from published papers. Where possible, we have utilized the same data set in more than one topic to reflect the reality of data analysis, which is rarely restricted to a single technique or approach. Although we believe that formulae should be provided and the logic of the approach explained as an aid to understanding, we have avoided showing the details of complex calculations—most readers will have access to computers and are unlikely to perform any but the simplest calculations by hand.

We consider that it is particularly important for the reader to be able to interpret output from a computer package. We have therefore chosen, where applicable, to show results using extracts from computer output. In some instances, when we believe individuals may have difficulty with its interpretation, we have included (Appendix C) and annotated the complete computer output from an analysis of a data set. There are many statistical packages in common use; to give the reader an indication of how output can vary, we have not restricted the output to a particular package and have, instead, used three well known ones: SAS, SPSS and STATA.

We wish to thank everyone who has helped us by providing data for the examples. We are particularly grateful to Richard Morris, Fiona Lampe and Shak Hajat, who read the entire book, and Abul Basar who read a substantial portion of it, all of whom made invaluable comments and suggestions. Naturally, we take full responsibility for any remaining errors in the text or examples.

It remains only to thank those who have lived and worked with us and our commitment to this project — Mike, Gerald, Nina, Andrew, Karen, and Diane. They have shown tolerance and understanding, particularly in the months leading to its completion, and have given us the opportunity to concentrate on this venture and bring it to fruition.

1 Types of data

Data and statistics

The purpose of most studies is to collect **data** to obtain information about a particular area of research. Our data comprise **observations** on one or more variables; any quantity that varies is termed a **variable**. For example, we may collect basic clinical and demographic information on patients with a particular illness. The variables of interest may include the sex, age and height of the patients.

Our data are usually obtained from a **sample** of individuals which represents the **population** of interest. Our aim is to condense these data in a meaningful way and extract useful information from them. **Statistics** encompasses the methods of collecting, summarizing, analysing and drawing conclusions from the data: we use statistical techniques to achieve our aim.

Data may take many different forms. We need to know what form every variable takes before we can make a decision regarding the most appropriate statistical methods to use. Each variable and the resulting data will be one of two types: **categorical** or **numerical** (Fig. 1.1).

Categorical (qualitative) data

These occur when each individual can only belong to one of a number of distinct categories of the variable.

• **Nominal data**—the categories are not ordered but simply have names. Examples include blood group (A, B, AB, and O) and marital status (married/widowed/single etc.). In this case there is no reason to suspect that being married is any better (or worse) than being single!

• **Ordinal data**—the categories are ordered in some way. Examples include disease staging systems (advanced, moderate, mild, none) and degree of pain (severe, moderate, mild, none).

A categorical variable is **binary** or **dichotomous** when there are only two possible categories. Examples include 'Yes/No', 'Dead/Alive' or 'Patient has disease/Patient does not have disease'.

Numerical (quantitative) data

These occur when the variable takes some numerical value. We can subdivide numerical data into two types.

• **Discrete data**—occur when the variable can only take certain whole numerical values. These are often counts of numbers of events, such as the number of visits to a GP in a year or the number of episodes of illness in an individual over the last five years.

• **Continuous data**—occur when there is no limitation on the values that the variable can take, e.g. weight or height, other than that which restricts us when we make the measurement.

Distinguishing between data types

We often use very different statistical methods depending on whether the data are categorical or numerical. Although the distinction between categorical and numerical data is usually clear, in some situations it may become blurred. For example, when we have a variable with a large number of ordered categories (e.g. a pain scale with seven categories), it may be difficult to distinguish it from a discrete numerical variable. The distinction between discrete and continuous numerical data may be even less clear, although in general this will have little impact on the results of most analyses. Age is an example of a variable that is often treated as discrete even though it is truly continuous. We usually refer to 'age at last birthday' rather than 'age', and therefore, a woman who reports being 30 may have just had her 30th birthday, or may be just about to have her 31st birthday.

Do not be tempted to record numerical data as categorical at the outset (e.g. by recording only the range within which each patient's age falls into rather than his/her actual age) as important information is often lost. It is simple to convert numerical data to categorical data once they have been collected.

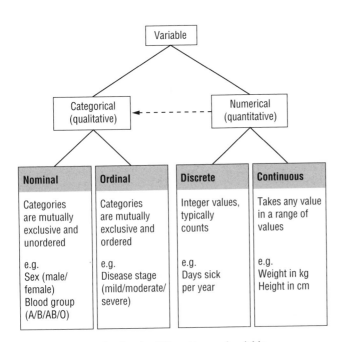

Fig. 1.1 Diagram showing the different types of variable.

Derived data

We may encounter a number of other types of data in the medical field. These include:

- **Percentages** — These may arise when considering improvements in patients following treatment, e.g. a patient's lung function (forced expiratory volume in 1 second, FEV1) may increase by 24% following treatment with a new drug. In this case, it is the level of improvement, rather than the absolute value, which is of interest.

- **Ratios** or **quotients** — Occasionally you may encounter the ratio or quotient of two variables. For example, body mass index (BMI), calculated as an individual's weight (kg) divided by his/her height squared (m^2) is often used to assess whether he/she is over- or under-weight.

- **Rates** — Disease rates, in which the number of disease events is divided by the time period under consideration, are common in epidemiological studies (Topic 12).

- **Scores** — We sometimes use an arbitrary value, i.e. a score, when we cannot measure a quantity. For example, a series of responses to questions on quality of life may be summed to give some overall quality of life score on each individual.

All these variables can be treated as continuous variables for most analyses. Where the variable is derived using more than one value (e.g. the numerator and denominator of a percentage), it is important to record all of the values used. For example, a 10% improvement in a marker following treatment may have different clinical relevance depending on the level of the marker before treatment.

Censored data

We may come across **censored** data in situations illustrated by the following examples.

- If we measure laboratory values using a tool that can only detect levels above a certain cut-off value, then any values below this cut-off will not be detected. For example, when measuring virus levels, those below the limit of detectability will often be reported as 'undetectable' even though there may be some virus in the sample.

- We may encounter censored data when following patients in a trial in which, for example, some patients withdraw from the trial before the trial has ended. This type of data is discussed in more detail in Topic 41.

2 Data entry

When you carry out any study you will almost always need to enter the data into a computer package. Computers are invaluable for improving the accuracy and speed of data collection and analysis, making it easy to check for errors, producing graphical summaries of the data and generating new variables. It is worth spending some time planning data entry—this may save considerable effort at later stages.

Formats for data entry

There are a number of ways in which data can be entered and stored on a computer. Most statistical packages allow you to enter data directly. However, the limitation of this approach is that often you cannot move the data to another package. A simple alternative is to store the data in either a spreadsheet or database package. Unfortunately, their statistical procedures are often limited, and it will usually be necessary to output the data into a specialist statistical package to carry out analyses.

A more flexible approach is to have your data available as an **ASCII** or **text** file. Once in an ASCII format, the data can be read by most packages. ASCII format simply consists of rows of text that you can view on a computer screen. Usually, each variable in the file is separated from the next by some **delimiter**, often a space or a comma. This is known as **free format**.

The simplest way of entering data in ASCII format is to type the data directly in this format using either a word processing or editing package. Alternatively, data stored in spreadsheet packages can be saved in ASCII format. Using either approach, it is customary for each row of data to correspond to a different individual in the study, and each column to correspond to a different variable, although it may be necessary to go on to subsequent rows if a large number of variables is collected on each individual.

Planning data entry

When collecting data in a study you will often need to use a form or questionnaire for recording data. If these are designed carefully, they can reduce the amount of work that has to be done when entering the data. Generally, these forms/questionnaires include a series of boxes in which the data are recorded—it is usual to have a separate box for each possible digit of the response.

Categorical data

Some statistical packages have problems dealing with non-numerical data. Therefore, you may need to assign numerical codes to categorical data before entering the data on to the computer. For example, you may choose to assign the codes of 1, 2, 3 and 4 to categories of 'no pain', 'mild pain', 'moderate pain' and 'severe pain', respectively. These codes can be added to the forms when collecting the data. For binary data, e.g. yes/no answers, it is often convenient to assign the codes 1 (e.g. for 'yes') and 0 (for 'no').

- **Single-coded** variables—there is only one possible answer to a question, e.g. 'is the patient dead?' It is not possible to answer both 'yes' and 'no' to this question.
- **Multi-coded** variables—more than one answer is possible for each respondent. For example, 'what symptoms has this patient experienced?' In this case, an individual may have experienced any of a number of symptoms. There are two ways to deal with this type of data depending upon which of the two following situations applies.
  - **There are only a few possible symptoms, and individuals may have experienced many of them.** A number of different binary variables can be created, which correspond to whether the patient has answered yes or no to the presence of each possible symptom. For example, 'did the patient have a cough?' 'Did the patient have a sore throat?'
  - **There are a very large number of possible symptoms but each patient is expected to suffer from only a few of them.** A number of different nominal variables can be created; each successive variable allows you to name a symptom suffered by the patient. For example, 'what was the first symptom the patient suffered?' 'What was the second symptom?' You will need to decide in advance the maximum number of symptoms you think a patient is likely to have suffered.

Numerical data

Numerical data should be entered with the same precision as they are measured, and the unit of measurement should be consistent for all observations on a variable. For example, weight should be recorded in kilograms or in pounds, but not both interchangeably.

Multiple forms per patient

Sometimes, information is collected on the same patient on more than one occasion. It is important that there is some unique identifier (e.g. a serial number) relating to the individual that will enable you to link all of the data from an individual in the study.

Problems with dates and times

Dates and times should be entered in a consistent manner, e.g. either as day/month/year or month/day/year, but not interchangeably. It is important to find out what format the statistical package can read.

Coding missing values

You should consider what you will do with missing values before you enter the data. In most cases you will need to use some symbol to represent a missing value. Statistical packages deal with missing values in different ways. Some use special characters (e.g. a full stop or asterisk) to indicate missing values, whereas others require you to define your own code for a missing value (commonly used values are 9, 999 or −99). The value that is chosen should be one that is not possible for that variable. For example, when entering a categorical variable with four categories (coded 1, 2, 3 and 4), you may choose the value 9 to represent missing values. However, if the variable is 'age of child' then a different code should be chosen. Missing data are discussed in more detail in Topic 3.

Example

Annotations:
- Nominal variables – no ordering to categories
- Discrete variable – can only take certain values in a range
- Multicoded variable – used to create four separate binary variables
- Error on questionnaire – some completed in kg, others in lb/oz.
- DATE
- Continuous variable
- Nominal
- Ordinal

Patient number	Bleeding deficiency	Sex of baby	Gestational age (weeks)	Interventions required during pregnancy				Apgar score	Weight of baby			Date of birth	Mothers age (years) at birth of child	Blood group	Frequency of bleeding gums
				Inhaled gas	IM Pethidine	IV Pethidine	Epidural		kg	lb	oz				
47	3	3	.	.	.	.	.	.	.	.	.	08/08/74	.	3	6
33	3	.	41	0	1	0	1	.	.	6	13	11/08/52	27.26	1	4
34	3	1	39	1	0	0	0	.	.	7	14	04/02/53	22.12	1	1
43	3	1	41	1	1	0	0	.	.	8	0	26/02/54	27.51	3	33
23	3	2	.	0	0	0	0	10/1-10/	11.19	.	.	29/12/65	36.58	1	3
49	3	3	.	.	.	.	.	.	.	.	.	09/08/57	.	1	5
51	3	3	.	.	.	.	.	.	.	.	.	21/06/51	.	3	5
20	2	.	41	0	1	0	0	.	.	7	12	15/08/96	25.61	3	3
64	4	.	.	1	1	0	0	.	.	.	.	10/11/51	24.61	3	2
27	3	1	14	1	0	0	0	ok	.	8	8	02/12/71	22.45	1	1
38	3	2	38	1	0	0	0	9/1-9/5	.	6	10	12/11/61	31.60	1	1
50	3	2	40	0	0	0	0	.	.	5	11	06/02/68	18.75	1	6
54	4	1	41	0	1	0	0	.	.	7	4	17/10/59	24.62	3	2
7	1	1	40	0	0	0	1	.	.	6	5	17/12/65	20.35	2	6
9	1	2	38	0	1	0	0	.	.	5	4	12/12/96	28.49	3	3
17	1	4	.	.	.	.	.	.	.	.	.	15/05/71	26.81	1	5
53	3	2	40	0	0	1	0	.	.	8	7	07/03/41	31.04	1	3
56	4	2	40	0	0	0	0	.	3.5	.	0	16/11/57	37.86	3	3
58	4	1	40	0	1	0	1	.	.	8	0	17/063/47	22.32	3	3
14	1	1	38	0	0	0	1	.	.	7	12	04/05/61	19.12	4	2

Legends:

Bleeding deficiency:
1=Haemophilia A
2=Haemophilia B
3=Von Willebrand's disease
4=FXI deficiency

Interventions:
0=No
1=Yes

Sex of baby:
1=Male
2=Female
3=Abortion
4=Still pregnant

Blood group:
1=O+ve
2=O−ve
3=A+ve
4=A−ve
5=B+ve
6=B−ve
7=AB+ve
8=AB−ve

Frequency of bleeding gums:
1=More than once a day
2=Once a day
3=Once a week
4=Once a month
5=Less frequently
6=Never

Fig. 2.1 Portion of a spreadsheet showing data collected on a sample of 64 women with inherited bleeding disorders.

As part of a study on the effect of inherited bleeding disorders on pregnancy and childbirth, data were collected on a sample of 64 women registered at a single haemophilia centre in London. The women were asked questions relating to their bleeding disorder and their first pregnancy (or their current pregnancy if they were pregnant for the first time on the date of interview). Fig. 2.1 shows the data from a small selection of the women after the data have been entered onto a spreadsheet, but before they have been checked for errors. The coding schemes for the categorical variables are shown at the bottom of Fig. 2.1. Each row of the spreadsheet represents a separate individual in the study; each column represents a different variable. Where the woman is still pregnant, the age of the woman at the time of birth has been calculated from the estimated date of the baby's delivery. Data relating to the live births are shown in Topic 34.

Data kindly provided by Dr R. A. Kadir, University Department of Obstetrics and Gynaecology, and Professor C. A. Lee, Haemophilia Centre and Haemostasis Unit, Royal Free Hospital, London.

3 Error checking and outliers

In any study there is always the potential for errors to occur in a data set, either at the outset when taking measurements, or when collecting, transcribing and entering the data onto a computer. It is hard to eliminate all of these errors. However, you can reduce the number of typing and transcribing errors by checking the data carefully once they have been entered. Simply scanning the data by eye will often identify values that are obviously wrong. In this topic we suggest a number of other approaches that you can use when checking data.

Typing errors

Typing mistakes are the most frequent source of errors when entering data. If the amount of data is small, then you can check the typed data set against the original forms/questionnaires to see whether there are any typing mistakes. However, this is time-consuming if the amount of data is large. It is possible to type the data in twice and compare the two data sets using a computer program. Any differences between the two data sets will reveal typing mistakes. Although this approach does not rule out the possibility that the same error has been incorrectly entered on both occasions, or that the value on the form/questionnaire is incorrect, it does at least minimize the number of errors. The disadvantage of this method is that it takes twice as long to enter the data, which may have major cost or time implications.

Error checking

- **Categorical data**—It is relatively easy to check categorical data, as the responses for each variable can only take one of a number of limited values. Therefore, values that are not allowable must be errors.
- **Numerical data**—Numerical data are often difficult to check but are prone to errors. For example, it is simple to transpose digits or to misplace a decimal point when entering numerical data. Numerical data can be **range checked**—that is, upper and lower limits can be specified for each variable. If a value lies outside this range then it is flagged up for further investigation.
- **Dates**—It is often difficult to check the accuracy of dates, although sometimes you may know that dates must fall within certain time periods. Dates can be checked to make sure that they are valid. For example, 30th February must be incorrect, as must any day of the month greater than 31, and any month greater than 12. Certain logical checks can also be applied. For example, a patient's date of birth should correspond to his/her age, and patients should usually have been born before entering the study (at least in most

studies). In addition, patients who have died should not appear for subsequent follow-up visits!

With all error checks, a value should only be corrected if there is evidence that a mistake has been made. You should not change values simply because they look unusual.

Handling missing data

There is always a chance that some data will be missing. If a very large proportion of the data is missing, then the results are unlikely to be reliable. The reasons why data are missing should always be investigated—if missing data tend to cluster on a particular variable and/or in a particular sub-group of individuals, then it may indicate that the variable is not applicable or has never been measured for that group of individuals. In the latter case, the group of individuals should be excluded from any analysis on that variable. It may be that the data are simply sitting on a piece of paper in someone's drawer and are yet to be entered!

Outliers

What are outliers?

Outliers are observations that are distinct from the main body of the data, and are incompatible with the rest of the data. These values may be genuine observations from individuals with very extreme levels of the variable. However, they may also result from typing errors, and so any suspicious values should be checked. It is important to detect whether there are outliers in the data set, as they may have a considerable impact on the results from some types of analyses.

For example, a woman who is 7 feet tall would probably appear as an outlier in most data sets. However, although this value is clearly very high, compared with the usual heights of women, it may be genuine and the woman may simply be very tall. In this case, you should investigate this value further, possibly checking other variables such as her age and weight, before making any decisions about the validity of the result. The value should only be changed if there really is evidence that it is incorrect.

Checking for outliers

A simple approach is to print the data and visually check them by eye. This is suitable if the number of observations is not too large and if the potential outlier is much lower or higher than the rest of the data. Range checking should also identify possible outliers. Alternatively, the data can be plotted in some way (Topic 4)—outliers can be clearly identified on histograms and scatter plots.

Handling outliers

It is important not to remove an individual from an analysis simply because his/her values are higher or lower than might be expected. However, the inclusion of outliers may affect the results when some statistical techniques are used. A simple approach is to repeat the analysis both including and excluding the value. If the results are similar, then the outlier does not have a great influence on the result. However, if the results change drastically, it is important to use appropriate methods that are not affected by outliers to analyse the data. These include the use of transformations (Topic 9) and non-parametric tests (Topic 17).

Example

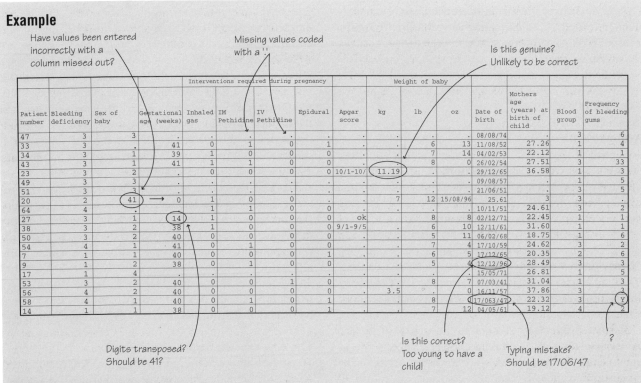

Fig. 3.1 Checking for errors in a data set.

After entering the data described in Topic 2, the data set is checked for errors. Some of the inconsistencies highlighted are simple data entry errors. For example, the code of '41' in the 'sex of baby' column is incorrect as a result of the sex information being missing for patient 20; the rest of the data for patient 20 had been entered in the incorrect columns. Others (e.g. unusual values in the gestational age and weight columns) are likely to be errors, but the notes should be checked before any decision is made, as these may reflect genuine outliers. In this case, the gestational age of patient number 27 was 41 weeks, and it was decided that a weight of 11.19 kg was incorrect. As it was not possible to find the correct weight for this baby, the value was entered as missing.

13

4 Displaying data graphically

One of the first things that you may wish to do when you have entered your data onto a computer is to summarize them in some way so that you can get a 'feel' for the data. This can be done by producing diagrams, tables or summary statistics (Topics 5 and 6). Diagrams are often powerful tools for conveying information about the data, for providing simple summary pictures, and for spotting outliers and trends before any formal analyses are performed.

One variable
Frequency distributions
An **empirical frequency distribution** of a variable relates each possible observation, class of observations (i.e. range of values) or category, as appropriate, to its observed **frequency** of occurrence. If we replace each frequency by a **relative frequency** (the percentage of the total frequency), we can compare frequency distributions in two or more groups of individuals.

Displaying frequency distributions
Once the frequencies (or relative frequencies) have been obtained for *categorical* or some *discrete numerical* data, these can be displayed visually.
- **Bar or column chart**—a separate horizontal or vertical bar is drawn for each category, its length being proportional to the frequency in that category. The bars are separated by small gaps to indicate that the data are categorical or discrete (Fig. 4.1a).
- **Pie chart**—a circular 'pie' is split into sections, one for each category, so that the area of each section is proportional to the frequency in that category (Fig. 4.1b).

It is often more difficult to display *continuous numerical* data, as the data may need to be summarized before being drawn. Commonly used diagrams include the following examples.
- **Histogram**—this is similar to a bar chart, but there should be no gaps between the bars as the data are continuous (Fig. 4.1d). The width of each bar of the histogram relates to a range of values for the variable. For example, the baby's weight (Fig. 4.1d) may be categorized into 1.75–1.99 kg, 2.00–2.24 kg, . . . , 4.25–4.49 kg. The area of the bar is proportional to the frequency in that range. Therefore, if one of the groups covers a wider range than the others, its base will be wider and height shorter to compensate. Usually, between five and 20 groups are chosen; the ranges should be narrow enough to illustrate patterns in the data, but should not be so narrow that they are the raw data. The histogram should be labelled carefully, to make it clear where the boundaries lie.

- **Dot plot**—each observation is represented by one dot on a horizontal (or vertical) line (Fig. 4.1e). This type of plot is very simple to draw, but can be cumbersome with large data sets. Often a summary measure of the data, such as the mean or median (Topic 5), is shown on the diagram. This plot may also be used for discrete data.
- **Stem-and-leaf plot**—This is a mixture of a diagram and a table; it looks similar to a histogram turned on its side, and is effectively the data values written in increasing order of size. It is usually drawn with a vertical **stem**, consisting of the first few digits of the values, arranged in order. Protruding from this stem are the **leaves**—i.e. the final digit of each of the ordered values, which are written horizontally (Fig. 4.2) in increasing numerical order.
- **Box plot** (often called a **box-and-whisker plot**)—This is a vertical or horizontal rectangle, with the ends of the rectangle corresponding to the upper and lower quartiles of the data values (Topic 6). A line drawn through the rectangle corresponds to the median value (Topic 5). Whiskers, starting at the ends of the rectangle, usually indicate minimum and maximum values but sometimes relate to particular percentiles, e.g. the 5th and 95th percentiles (Topic 6, Fig. 6.1). Outliers may be marked.

The 'shape' of the frequency distribution
The choice of the most appropriate statistical method will often depend on the shape of the distribution. The distribution of the data is usually **unimodal** in that it has a single 'peak'. Sometimes the distribution is **bimodal** (two peaks) or **uniform** (each value is equally likely and there are no peaks). When the distribution is unimodal, the main aim is to see where the majority of the data values lie, relative to the maximum and minimum values. In particular, it is important to assess whether the distribution is:
- **symmetrical**—centred around some mid-point, with one side being a mirror-image of the other (Fig. 5.1);
- **skewed to the right (positively skewed)**—a long tail to the right with one or a few high values. Such data are common in medical research (Fig. 5.2);
- **skewed to the left (negatively skewed)**—a long tail to the left with one or a few low values (Fig. 4.1d).

Two variables
If one variable is categorical, then separate diagrams showing the distribution of the second variable can be drawn for each of the categories. Other plots suitable for such data include **clustered** or **segmented** bar or column charts (Fig. 4.1c).

If both of the variables are continuous or ordinal, then

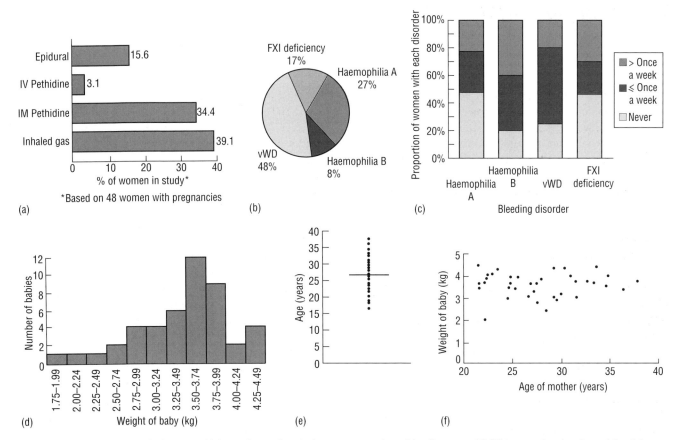

Fig. 4.1 A selection of graphical output which may be produced when summarizing the obstetric data in women with bleeding disorders (Topic 2). (a) **Bar chart** showing the percentage of women in the study who required pain relief from any of the listed interventions during labour. (b) **Pie chart** showing the percentage of women in the study with each bleeding disorder. (c) **Segmented column chart** showing the frequency with which women with different bleeding disorders experience bleeding gums. (d) **Histogram** showing the weight of the baby at birth. (e) **Dot-plot** showing the mother's age at the time of the baby's birth, with the median age marked as a horizontal line. (f) **Scatter diagram** showing the relationship between the mother's age at delivery (on the horizontal or *x*-axis) and the weight of the baby (on the vertical or *y*-axis).

the relationship between the two can be illustrated using a **scatter diagram** (Fig. 4.1f). This plots one variable against the other in a two-way diagram. One variable is usually termed the *x* variable and is represented on the horizontal axis. The second variable, known as the *y* variable, is plotted on the vertical axis.

Identifying outliers using graphical methods

We can often use single variable data displays to identify outliers. For example, a very long tail on one side of a histogram may indicate an outlying value. However, outliers may sometimes only become apparent when considering the relationship between two variables. For example, a weight of 55 kg would not be unusual for a woman who was 1.6 m tall, but would be unusually low if the woman's height was 1.9 m.

3	1.0	04
665	1.1	39
53	1.2	99
9751	1.3	1135677999
955410	1.4	0148
987655	1.5	00338899
9531100	1.6	0001355
731	1.7	00114569
99843110	1.8	6
654400	1.9	01
6	2.0	
7	2.1	19
10	2.2	
Beclomethasone dipropionate		Placebo

Fig. 4.2 Stem-and-leaf plot showing the FEV1 (litres) in children receiving inhaled beclomethasone dipropionate or placebo (Topic 21).

15

5 Describing data (1): the 'average'

Summarizing data

It is very difficult to have any 'feeling' for a set of numerical measurements unless we can summarize the data in a meaningful way. A diagram (Topic 4) is often a useful starting point. We can also condense the information by providing measures that describe the important characteristics of the data. In particular, if we have some perception of what constitutes a representative value, and if we know how widely scattered the observations are around it, then we can formulate an image of the data. The **average** is a general term for a measure of **location**; it describes a typical measurement. We devote this topic to averages, the most common being the mean and median (Table 5.1). We introduce you to measures that describe the scatter or **spread** of the observations in Topic 6.

The arithmetic mean

The **arithmetic mean**, often simply called the mean, of a set of values is calculated by adding up all the values and dividing this sum by the number of values in the set.

It is useful to be able to summarize this verbal description by an algebraic formula. Using mathematical notation, we write our set of n observations of a variable, x, as x_1, x_2, $x_3, \ldots, x_n$. For example, x might represent an individual's height (cm), so that x_1 represents the height of the first individual, and x_i the height of the ith individual, etc. We can write the formula for the arithmetic mean of the observations, written $\bar{x}$ and pronounced 'x bar', as:

$$\bar{x} = \frac{x_1 + x_2 + x_3 + \ldots + x_n}{n}$$

Using mathematical notation, we can shorten this to:

$$\bar{x} = \frac{\sum_{i=1}^{n} x_i}{n}$$

where Σ (the Greek uppercase 'sigma') means 'the sum of', and the sub- and super-scripts on the Σ indicate that we sum the values from $i = 1$ to n. This is often further abbreviated to

$$\bar{x} = \frac{\sum x_i}{n} \quad \text{or to} \quad \bar{x} = \frac{\sum x}{n}$$

The median

If we arrange our data in order of magnitude, starting with the smallest value and ending with the largest value, then the **median** is the middle value of this ordered set. The median divides the ordered values into two halves, with an equal number of values both above and below it.

It is easy to calculate the median if the number of observations, n, is **odd**. It is the $(n + 1)/2$th observation in the ordered set. So, for example, if $n = 11$, then the median is the $(11 + 1)/2 = 12/2 = 6$th observation in the ordered set. If n is

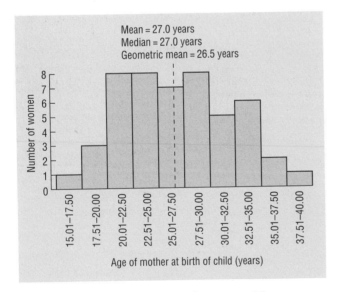

Fig. 5.1 The mean, median and geometric mean age of the women in the study described in Topic 2 at the time of the baby's birth. As the distribution of age appears reasonably symmetrical, the three measures of the 'average' all give similar values, as indicated by the dotted line.

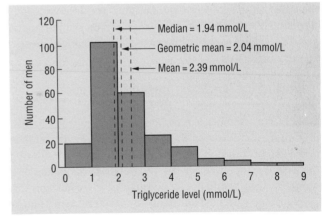

Fig. 5.2 The mean, median and geometric mean triglyceride level in a sample of 232 men who developed heart disease (Topic 19). As the distribution of triglyceride is skewed to the right, the mean gives a higher 'average' than either the median or geometric mean.

even then, strictly, there is no median. However, we usually calculate it as the arithmetic mean of the two middle observations in the ordered set [i.e. the $n/2$th and the $(n/2 + 1)$th]. So, for example, if $n = 20$, the median is the arithmetic mean of the $20/2 = 10$th and the $(20/2 + 1) = (10 + 1) = 11$th observations in the ordered set.

The median is similar to the mean if the data are symmetrical (Fig. 5.1), less than the mean if the data are skewed to the right (Fig. 5.2), and greater than the mean if the data are skewed to the left.

The mode

The **mode** is the value that occurs most frequently in a data set; if the data are continuous, we usually group the data and calculate the modal group. Some data sets do not have a mode because each value only occurs once. Sometimes, there is more than one mode; this is when two or more values occur the same number of times, and the frequency of occurrence of each of these values is greater than that of any other value. We rarely use the mode as a summary measure.

The geometric mean

The arithmetic mean is an inappropriate summary measure of location if our data are skewed. If the data are skewed to the right, we can produce a distribution that is more symmetrical if we take the logarithm (to base 10 or to base e) of each value of the variable in this data set (Topic 9). The arithmetic mean of the log values is a measure of location for the transformed data. To obtain a measure that has the same units as the original observations, we have to back-transform (i.e. take the antilog of) the mean of the log data; we call this the **geometric mean**. Provided the distribution of the log data is approximately symmetrical, the geometric mean is similar to the median and less than the mean of the raw data (Fig. 5.2).

The weighted mean

We use a **weighted mean** when certain values of the variable of interest, x, are more important than others. We attach a weight, w_i, to each of the values, x_i, in our sample, to reflect this importance. If the values $x_1, x_2, x_3, \ldots, x_n$ have corresponding weights $w_1, w_2, w_3, \ldots, w_n$ the weighted arithmetic mean is:

$$\frac{w_1 x_1 + w_2 x_2 + \ldots + w_n x_n}{w_1 + w_2 + \ldots + w_n} = \frac{\sum w_i x_i}{\sum w_i}$$

For example, suppose we are interested in determining the average length of stay of hospitalized patients in a district, and we know the average discharge time for patients in every hospital. To take account of the amount of information provided, one approach might be to take each weight as the number of patients in the associated hospital.

The weighted mean and the arithmetic mean are identical if each weight is equal to one.

Table 5.1 Advantages and disadvantages of averages.

Type of average	Advantages	Disadvantages
Mean	• Uses all the data values • Algebraically defined and so mathematically manageable • Known sampling distribution (Topic 9)	• Distorted by outliers • Distorted by skewed data
Median	• Not distorted by outliers • Not distorted by skewed data	• Ignores most of the information • Not algebraically defined • Complicated sampling distribution
Mode	• Easily determined for categorical data	• Ignores most of the information • Not algebraically defined • Unknown sampling distribution
Geometric mean	• Before back-transformation, it has the same advantages as the mean • Appropriate for right skewed data	• Only appropriate if the log transformation produces a symmetrical distribution
Weighted mean	• Same advantages as the mean • Ascribes relative importance to each observation • Algebraically defined	• Weights must be known or estimated

6 Describing data (2): the 'spread'

Summarizing data

If we are able to provide two summary measures of a continuous variable, one that gives an indication of the 'average' value and the other that describes the 'spread' of the observations, then we have condensed the data in a meaningful way. We explained how to choose an appropriate average in Topic 5. We devote this topic to a discussion of the most common measures of **spread** (**dispersion** or **variability**) which are compared in Table 6.1.

The range

The **range** is the difference between the largest and smallest observations in the data set; you may find these two values quoted instead of their difference. Note that the range provides a misleading measure of spread if there are outliers (Topic 3).

Ranges derived from percentiles
What are percentiles?

Suppose we arrange our data in order of magnitude, starting with the smallest value of the variable, x, and ending with the largest value. The value of x that has 1% of the observations in the ordered set lying below it (and 99% of the observations lying above it) is called the first **percentile**. The value of x that has 2% of the observations lying below it is called the second percentile, and so on. The values of x that divide the ordered set into 10 equally sized groups, that is the 10th, 20th, 30th, . . . , 90th percentiles, are called

deciles. The values of x that divide the ordered set into four equally sized groups, that is the 25th, 50th, and 75th percentiles, are called **quartiles**. The 50th percentile is the **median** (Topic 5).

Using percentiles

We can obtain a measure of spread that is not influenced by outliers by excluding the extreme values in the data set, and determining the range of the remaining observations. The **interquartile range** is the difference between the first and the third quartiles, i.e. between the 25th and 75th percentiles (Fig. 6.1). It contains the central 50% of the observations in the ordered set, with 25% of the observations lying below its lower limit, and 25% of them lying above its upper limit. The **interdecile range** contains the central 80% of the observations, i.e. those lying between the 10th and 90th percentiles. Often we use the range that contains the central 95% of the observations, i.e. it excludes 2.5% of the observations above its upper limit and 2.5% below its lower limit (Fig. 6.1). We may use this interval, provided it is calculated from enough values of the variable in healthy individuals, to diagnose disease. It is then called the **reference interval**, **reference range** or **normal range** (Topic 35).

The variance

One way of measuring the spread of the data is to determine the extent to which each observation deviates from the arithmetic mean. Clearly, the larger the deviations, the

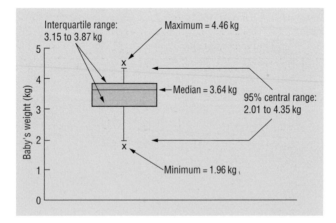

Fig. 6.1 A box-and-whisker plot of the baby's weight at birth (Topic 2). This figure illustrates the median, the interquartile range, the range that contains the central 95% of the observations and the maximum and minimum values.

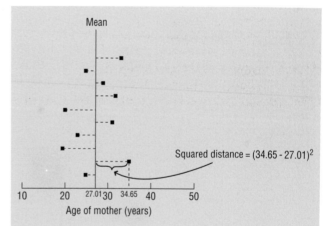

Fig. 6.2 Diagram showing the spread of selected values of the mother's age at the time of baby's birth (Topic 2) around the mean value. The variance is calculated by adding up the squared distances between each point and the mean, and dividing by $(n-1)$.

greater the variability of the observations. However, we cannot use the mean of these deviations as a measure of spread because the positive differences exactly cancel out the negative differences. We overcome this problem by squaring each deviation, and finding the mean of these squared deviations (Fig. 6.2); we call this the **variance**. If we have a sample of n observations, $x_1, x_2, x_3, \ldots, x_n$, whose mean is $\bar{x} = (\Sigma x_i)/n$, we calculate the variance, usually denoted by s^2, of these observations as:

$$s^2 = \frac{\sum (x_i - \bar{x})^2}{n-1}$$

We can see that this is not quite the same as the arithmetic mean of the squared deviations because we have divided by $n-1$ instead of n. The reason for this is that we almost always rely on *sample* data in our investigations (Topic 10). It can be shown theoretically that we obtain a better sample estimate of the population variance if we divide by $n-1$.

The units of the variance are the square of the units of the original observations, e.g. if the variable is weight measured in kg, the units of the variance are kg^2.

The standard deviation

The **standard deviation** is the square root of the variance. In a sample of n observations, it is:

$$s = \sqrt{\frac{\sum (x_i - \bar{x})^2}{n-1}}$$

We can think of the standard deviation as a sort of average of the deviations of the observations from the mean. It is evaluated in the same units as the raw data.

If we divide the standard deviation by the mean and express this quotient as a percentage, we obtain the **coefficient of variation**. It is a measure of spread that is independent of the units of measurement, but it has theoretical disadvantages so is not favoured by statisticians.

Variation within- and between-subjects

If we take repeated measurements of a continuous variable on an individual, then we expect to observe some variation (**intra-** or **within-subject** variability) in the responses on that individual. This may be because a given individual does not always respond in exactly the same way and/or because of measurement error. However, the variation within an individual is usually less than the variation obtained when we take a single measurement on every individual in a group (**inter-** or **between-subject** variability). For example, a 17-year-old boy has a lung vital capacity that ranges between 3.60 and 3.87 litres when the measurement is repeated 10 times; the values for single measurements on 10 boys of the same age lie between 2.98 and 4.33 litres. These concepts are important in study design (Topic 13).

Table 6.1 Advantages and disadvantages of measures of spread.

Measure of spread	Advantages	Disadvantages
Range	• Easily determined	• Uses only two observations • Distorted by outliers • Tends to increase with increasing sample size
Ranges based on percentiles	• Unaffected by outliers • Independent of sample size • Appropriate for skewed data	• Clumsy to calculate • Cannot be calculated for small samples • Uses only two observations • Not algebraically defined
Variance	• Uses every observation • Algebraically defined	• Units of measurement are the square of the units of the raw data • Sensitive to outliers • Inappropriate for skewed data
Standard deviation	• Same advantages as the variance • Units of measurement are the same as those of the raw data • Easily interpreted	• Sensitive to outliers • Inappropriate for skewed data

7 Theoretical distributions (1): the Normal distribution

In Topic 4 we showed how to create an **empirical frequency distribution** of the observed data. This contrasts with a theoretical **probability distribution**, which is described by a mathematical model. When our empirical distribution approximates a particular probability distribution, we can use our theoretical knowledge of that distribution to answer questions about the data. This often requires the evaluation of probabilities.

Understanding probability

Probability measures uncertainty; it lies at the heart of statistical theory. A probability measures the chance of a given event occurring. It is a positive number that lies between zero and one. If it is equal to zero, then the event *cannot* occur. If it is equal to one, then the event *must* occur. The probability of the **complementary** event (the event *not* occurring) is one minus the probability of the event occurring. We discuss **conditional probability**, the probability of an event, given that another event has occurred, in Topic 42.

We can calculate a probability using various approaches.
- **Subjective** — our personal degree of belief that the event will occur (e.g. that the world will come to an end in the year 2050).
- **Frequentist** — the proportion of times the event would occur if we were to repeat the experiment a large number of times (e.g. the number of times we would get a 'head' if we tossed a fair coin 1000 times).
- **A priori** — this requires knowledge of the theoretical *model*, called the **probability distribution**, which describes the probabilities of all possible outcomes of the 'experiment'. For example, genetic theory allows us to describe the probability distribution for eye colour in a baby born to a blue-eyed woman and brown-eyed man by initially specifying all possible genotypes of eye colour in the baby and their probabilities.

The rules of probability

We can use the rules of probability to add and multiply probabilities.
- **The addition rule** — if two events, A and B, are *mutually exclusive* (i.e. each event precludes the other), then the probability that either one or the other occurs is equal to the sum of their probabilities.

$$\text{Prob}(A \text{ } or \text{ } B) = \text{Prob}(A) + \text{Prob}(B)$$

e.g. if the probabilities that an adult patient in a particular dental practice has no missing teeth, some missing teeth or is edentulous (i.e. has no teeth) are 0.67, 0.24 and 0.09,

respectively, then the probability that a patient has some teeth is $0.67 + 0.24 = 0.91$.
- **The multiplication rule** — if two events, A and B, are *independent* (i.e. the occurrence of one event is not contingent on the other), then the probability that both events occur is equal to the product of the probability of each:
$\text{Prob}(A \text{ } and \text{ } B) = \text{Prob}(A) \times \text{Prob}(B)$ e.g. if two unrelated patients are waiting in the dentist's surgery, the probability that both of them have no missing teeth is $0.67 \times 0.67 = 0.45$.

Probability distributions: the theory

A **random variable** is a quantity that can take any one of a set of mutually exclusive values with a given probability. A **probability distribution** shows the probabilities of all possible values of the random variable. It is a theoretical distribution that is expressed mathematically, and has a mean and variance that are analogous to those of an empirical distribution. Each probability distribution is defined by certain **parameters**, which are summary measures (e.g. mean, variance) characterizing that distribution (i.e. knowledge of them allows the distribution to be fully described). These parameters are estimated in the sample by relevant **statistics**. Depending on whether the random variable is discrete or continuous, the probability distribution can be either discrete or continuous.
- **Discrete** (e.g. Binomial, Poisson) — we can derive probabilities corresponding to every possible value of the random variable. *The sum of all such probabilities is one*.
- **Continuous** (e.g. Normal, Chi-squared, t and F) — we can only derive the probability of the random variable, x, taking values in certain ranges (because there are infinitely many values of x). If the horizontal axis represents the values of x,

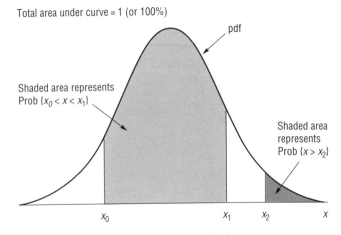

Total area under curve = 1 (or 100%)

Shaded area represents Prob $\{x_0 < x < x_1\}$

Shaded area represents Prob $\{x > x_2\}$

pdf

Fig. 7.1 The probability density function, pdf, of x.

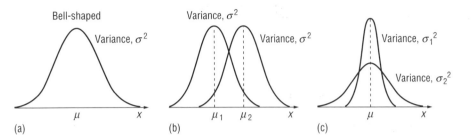

Fig. 7.2 The probability density function of the Normal distribution of the variable, x. (a) Symmetrical about mean, μ: variance = σ^2. (b) Effect of changing mean ($\mu_2 > \mu_1$). (c) Effect of changing variance ($\sigma_1^2 < \sigma_2^2$).

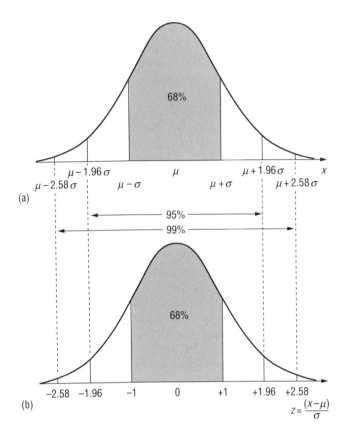

Fig. 7.3 Areas (percentages of total probability) under the curve for (a) Normal distribution of x, with mean μ and variance σ^2, and (b) Standard Normal distribution of z.

we can draw a curve from the equation of the distribution (the **probability density function**); it resembles an empirical relative frequency distribution (Topic 4). *The total area under the curve is one*; this area represents the probability of all possible events. The probability that x lies between two limits is equal to the area under the curve between these values (Fig. 7.1). For convenience, tables (Appendix A) have been produced to enable us to evaluate probabilities of interest for commonly used continuous probability distributions. These are particularly useful in the context of confidence intervals (Topic 11) and hypothesis testing (Topic 17).

The Normal (Gaussian) distribution

One of the most important distributions in statistics is the **Normal distribution**. Its probability density function (Fig. 7.2) is:

- completely described by two parameters, the *mean* (μ) and the *variance* (σ^2);
- bell-shaped (unimodal);
- symmetrical about its mean;
- shifted to the right if the mean is increased and to the left if the mean is decreased (assuming constant variance);
- flattened as the variance is increased but becomes more peaked as the variance is decreased (for a fixed mean).

Additional properties are that:

- the mean and median of a Normal distribution are equal;
- the probability (Fig. 7.3a) that a Normally distributed random variable, x, with mean, μ, and standard deviation, σ, lies between:

$(\mu - \sigma)$ and $(\mu + \sigma)$ is 0.68

$(\mu - 1.96\sigma)$ and $(\mu + 1.96\sigma)$ is 0.95

$(\mu - 2.58\sigma)$ and $(\mu + 2.58\sigma)$ is 0.99

These intervals may be used to define **reference intervals** (Topics 6 and 35).

We show how to assess Normality in Topic 32.

The Standard Normal distribution

There are infinitely many Normal distributions depending on the values of μ and σ. The Standard Normal distribution (Fig. 7.3b) is a particular Normal distribution for which probabilities have been tabulated (Appendix A1, A4).

- The Standard Normal distribution has a **mean of zero** and a **variance of one**.
- If the random variable, x, has a Normal distribution with mean, μ, and variance, σ^2, then the **Standardized Normal Deviate (SND)**, $z = \dfrac{x - \mu}{\sigma}$, is a random variable that has a Standard Normal distribution.

8 Theoretical distributions (2): other distributions

Some words of comfort

Do not worry if you find the theory underlying probability distributions complex. Our experience demonstrates that you want to know only when and how to use these distributions. We have therefore outlined the essentials, and omitted the equations that define the probability distributions. You will find that you only need to be familiar with the basic ideas, the terminology and, perhaps (although infrequently in this computer age), know how to refer to the tables.

More continuous probability distributions

These distributions are based on continuous random variables. Often it is not a measurable variable that follows such a distribution, but a statistic derived from the variable. The total area under the probability density function represents the probability of all possible outcomes, and is equal to one (Topic 7). We discussed the Normal distribution in Topic 7; other common distributions are described in this topic.

The *t*-distribution (Appendix A2, Fig. 8.1)

• Derived by W.S. Gossett, who published under the pseudonym 'Student', it is often called Student's *t*-distribution.

• The parameter that characterizes the *t*-distribution is the **degrees of freedom**, so we can draw the probability density function if we know the equation of the *t*-distribution and its degrees of freedom. We discuss degrees of freedom in Topic 11; note that they are often closely affiliated to sample size.

• Its shape is similar to that of the Standard Normal distribution, but it is more spread out with longer tails. Its shape approaches Normality as the degrees of freedom increase.

• It is particularly useful for calculating confidence intervals for and testing hypotheses about one or two means (Topics 19–21).

The Chi-squared (χ^2) distribution (Appendix A3, Fig. 8.2)

• It is a right skewed distribution taking positive values.

• It is characterized by its **degrees of freedom** (Topic 11).

• Its shape depends on the degrees of freedom; it becomes more symmetrical and approaches Normality as they increase.

• It is particularly useful for analysing categorical data (Topics 23–25).

The *F*-distribution (Appendix A5)

• It is skewed to the right.

• It is defined by a ratio. The distribution of a ratio of two estimated variances calculated from Normal data approximates the *F*-distribution.

• The two parameters which characterize it are the **degrees of freedom** (Topic 11) of the numerator and the denominator of the ratio.

• The *F*-distribution is particularly useful for comparing two variances (Topic 18), and more than two means using the analysis of variance (ANOVA) (Topic 22).

The Lognormal distribution

• It is the probability distribution of a random variable whose log (to base 10 or *e*) follows the Normal distribution.

• It is highly skewed to the right (Fig. 8.3a).

• If, when we take logs of our raw data that are skewed to the right, we produce an empirical distribution that is

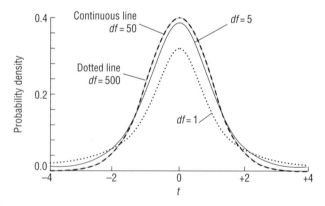

Fig. 8.1 *t*-distributions with degrees of freedom (*df*) = 1, 5, 50, and 500.

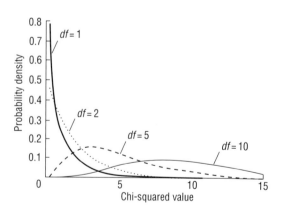

Fig. 8.2 Chi-squared distributions with degrees of freedom (*df*) = 1, 2, 5, and 10.

nearly Normal (Fig. 8.3b), our data approximate the Lognormal distribution.
- Many variables in medicine follow a Lognormal distribution. We can use the properties of the Normal distribution (Topic 7) to make inferences about these variables after transforming the data by taking logs.
- If a data set has a Lognormal distribution, we use the geometric mean (Topic 5) as a summary measure of location.

Discrete probability distributions

The random variable that defines the probability distribution is discrete. The sum of the probabilities of all possible mutually exclusive events is one.

The Binomial distribution

- Suppose, in a given situation, there are only two outcomes, 'success' and 'failure'. For example, we may be interested in whether a woman conceives (a success) or does not conceive (a failure) after in-vitro fertilization (IVF). If we look at $n = 100$ unrelated women undergoing IVF (each with the same probability of conceiving), the Binomial random variable is the observed number of conceptions (successes). Often this concept is explained in terms of n independent repetitions of a trial (e.g. 100 tosses of a coin) in which the outcome is either success (e.g. head) or failure.
- The two parameters that describe the Binomial distribution are n, the number of individuals in the sample (or repetitions of a trial) and π, the true probability of success for each individual (or in each trial).

- Its **mean** (the value for the random variable that we *expect* if we look at n individuals, or repeat the trial n times) is $n\pi$. Its **variance** is $n\pi(1 - \pi)$.
- When n is small, the distribution is skewed to the right if $\pi < 0.5$ and to the left if $\pi > 0.5$. The distribution becomes more symmetrical as the sample size increases (Fig. 8.4) and approximates the Normal distribution if both $n\pi$ and $n(1 - \pi)$ are greater than 5.
- We can use the properties of the Binomial distribution when making inferences about **proportions**. In particular we often use the Normal approximation to the Binomial distribution when analysing proportions.

The Poisson distribution

- The Poisson random variable is the **count** of the number of events that occur independently and randomly in time or space at some average rate, μ. For example, the number of hospital admissions per day typically follows the Poisson distribution. We can use our knowledge of the Poisson distribution to calculate the probability of a certain number of admissions on any particular day.
- The parameter that describes the Poisson distribution is the **mean**, i.e. the average rate, μ.
- The **mean** equals the **variance** in the Poisson distribution.
- It is a right skewed distribution if the mean is small, but becomes more symmetrical as the mean increases, when it approximates a Normal distribution.

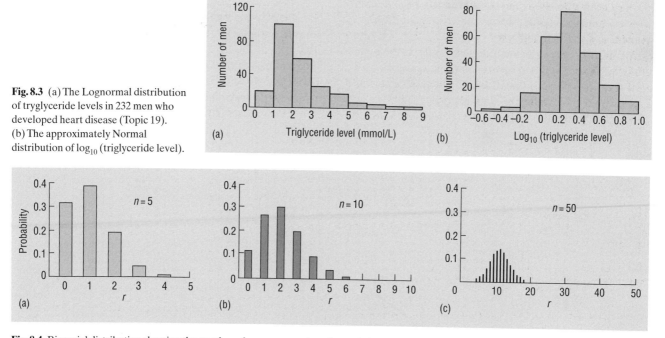

Fig. 8.3 (a) The Lognormal distribution of tryglyceride levels in 232 men who developed heart disease (Topic 19). (b) The approximately Normal distribution of $\log_{10}$ (triglyceride level).

Fig. 8.4 Binomial distribution showing the number of successes, r, when the probability of success is $\pi = 0.20$ for sample sizes (a) $n = 5$, (b) $n = 10$, and (c) $n = 50$. (N.B. in Topic 23, the observed seroprevalence of HHV-8 was $p = 0.187 \approx 0.2$, and the sample size was 271: the proportion was assumed to follow a Normal distribution).

9 Transformations

Why transform?

The observations in our investigation may not comply with the requirements of the intended statistical analysis (Topic 32).

- A variable may not be Normally distributed, a **distributional** requirement for many different analyses.
- The spread of the observations in each of a number of groups may be different (constant variance is an assumption about a **parameter** in the comparison of means using the t-test and analysis of variance—Topics 21–22).
- Two variables may not be linearly related (**linearity** is an assumption in many regression analyses—Topics 27–31).

It is often helpful to **transform** our data to satisfy the assumptions underlying the proposed statistical techniques.

How do we transform?

We convert our raw data into transformed data by taking the same mathematical transformation of each observation. Suppose we have n observations $(y_1, y_2, \ldots, y_n)$ on a variable, y, and we decide that the log transformation is suitable. We take the log of each observation to produce $(\log y_1, \log y_2, \ldots, \log y_n)$. If we call the transformed variable, z, then $z_i = \log y_i$ for each i ($i = 1, 2, \ldots, n$), and our transformed data may be written $(z_1, z_2, \ldots, z_n)$.

We check that the transformation has achieved its purpose of producing a data set that satisfies the assumptions of the planned statistical analysis, and proceed to analyse the transformed data $(z_1, z_2, \ldots, z_n)$. We often back-transform any summary measures (such as the mean) to the original scale of measurement; the conclusions we draw from hypothesis tests (Topic 17) on the transformed data are applicable to the raw data.

Typical transformations

The logarithmic transformation, $z = \log y$

When log transforming data, we can choose to take logs either to base 10 ($\log_{10} y$, the 'common' log) or to base e ($\log_e y = \ln y$, the 'natural' or Naperian log), but must be consistent for a particular variable in a data set. Note that we cannot take the log of a negative number or of zero. The back-transformation of a log is called the antilog; the antilog of a Naperian log is the exponential, e.

- If y is skewed to the right, $z = \log y$ is often approximately **Normally distributed** (Fig. 9.1a). Then y has a Lognormal distribution (Topic 8).
- If there is an exponential relationship between y and another variable, x, so that the resulting curve bends upwards when y (on the vertical axis) is plotted against x (on the horizontal axis), then the relationship between $z = \log y$ and x is approximately **linear** (Fig. 9.1b).
- Suppose we have different groups of observations, each comprising measurements of a continuous variable, y. We may find that the groups that have the higher values of y also have larger variances. In particular, if the coefficient of variation (the standard deviation divided by the mean) of y is constant for all the groups, the log transformation, $z = \log y$, produces groups that have the **same variance** (Fig. 9.1c).

In medicine, the log transformation is frequently used because of its logical interpretation and because many variables have right-skewed distributions.

The square root transformation, $z = \sqrt{y}$

This transformation has properties that are similar to those of the log transformation, although the results after they

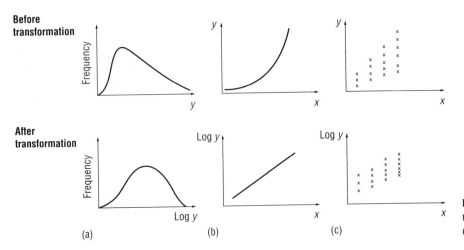

Before transformation

Frequency / y

y / x

y / x

After transformation

Frequency / $\log y$

$\log y$ / x

$\log y$ / x

(a)　　　(b)　　　(c)

Fig. 9.1 The effects of the logarithmic transformation. (a) Normalizing. (b) Linearizing. (c) Variance stabilizing.

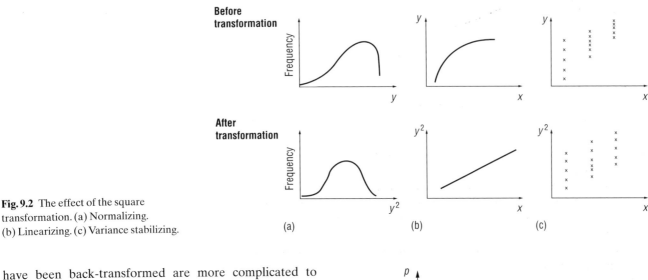

Fig. 9.2 The effect of the square transformation. (a) Normalizing. (b) Linearizing. (c) Variance stabilizing.

have been back-transformed are more complicated to interpret. In addition to its **Normalizing** and **linearizing** abilities, it is effective at **stabilizing variance** if the variance increases with increasing values of y, i.e. if the variance divided by the mean is constant. We apply the square root transformation if y is the count of a rare event occurring in time or space, i.e. it is a Poisson variable (Topic 8). Remember, we cannot take the square root of a negative number.

The reciprocal transformation, $z = 1/y$

We often apply the reciprocal transformation to survival times unless we are using special techniques for survival analysis (Topic 41). The reciprocal transformation has properties that are similar to those of the log transformation. In addition to its **Normalizing** and **linearizing** abilities, it is more effective at **stabilizing variance** than the log transformation if the variance increases very markedly with increasing values of y, i.e. if the variance divided by the (mean)^4 is constant. Note that we cannot take the reciprocal of zero.

The square transformation, $z = y^2$

The square transformation achieves the reverse of the log transformation.
• If y is skewed to the left, the distribution of $z = y^2$ is often approximately **Normal** (Fig. 9.2a).
• If the relationship between two variables, x and y, is such that a line curving downwards is produced when we plot y against x, then the relationship between $z = y^2$ and x is approximately **linear** (Fig. 9.2b).

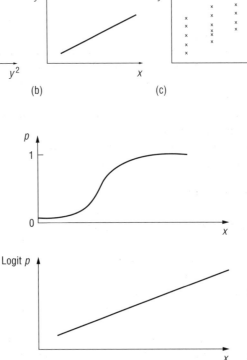

Fig. 9.3 The effect of the logit transformation on a sigmoid curve.

• If the variance of a continuous variable, y, tends to decrease as the value of y increases, then the square transformation, $z = y^2$, **stabilizes the variance** (Fig. 9.2c).

The logit (logistic) transformation, $z = \ln \dfrac{p}{1-p}$

This is the transformation we apply most often to each proportion, p, in a set of proportions. We cannot take the logit transformation if either $p = 0$ or $p = 1$ because the corresponding logit values are $-\infty$ and $+\infty$. One solution is to take p as $1/(2n)$ instead of 0, and as $\{1 - 1/(2n)\}$ instead of 1.

It **linearizes** a sigmoid curve (Fig. 9.3).

10 Sampling and sampling distributions

Why do we sample?

In statistics, a **population** represents the entire group of individuals in whom we are interested. Generally it is costly and labour-intensive to study the entire population and, in some cases, may be impossible because the population may be hypothetical (e.g. patients who may receive a treatment in the future). Therefore we collect data on a **sample** of individuals who we believe are **representative** of this population, and use them to draw conclusions (i.e. make **inferences**) about the population.

When we take a sample of the population, we have to recognize that the information in the sample may not fully reflect what is true in the population. We have introduced **sampling error** by studying only some of the population. In this topic we show how to use theoretical probability distributions (Topics 7 and 8) to quantify this error.

Obtaining a representative sample

Ideally, we aim for a **random sample**. A list of all individuals from the population is drawn up (the **sampling frame**), and individuals are selected randomly from this list, i.e. every possible sample of a given size in the population has an equal probability of being chosen. Sometimes, we may have difficulty in constructing this list or the costs involved may be prohibitive, and then we take a **convenience sample**. For example, when studying patients with a particular clinical condition, we may choose a single hospital, and investigate some or all of the patients with the condition in that hospital. Very occasionally, non-random schemes, such as **quota sampling** or **systematic sampling**, may be used. Although the statistical tests described in this book assume that individuals are selected for the sample **randomly**, the methods are generally reasonable as long as the sample is **representative** of the population.

Point estimates

We are often interested in the value of a **parameter** in the population (Topic 7), e.g. a mean or a proportion. Parameters are usually denoted by letters of the Greek alphabet. For example, we usually refer to the population mean as μ and the population standard deviation as σ. We estimate the value of the parameter using the data collected from the sample. This estimate is referred to as the **sample statistic** and is a **point estimate** of the parameter (i.e. it takes a single value) as distinct from an **interval estimate** (Topic 11) which takes a range of values.

Sampling variation

If we take repeated samples of the same size from a popula-

tion, it is unlikely that the estimates of the population parameter would be exactly the same in each sample. However, our estimates should all be close to the true value of the parameter in the population, and the estimates themselves should be similar to each other. By quantifying the variability of these estimates, we obtain information on the precision of our estimate and can thereby assess the sampling error. *In reality, we usually only take one sample from the population.* However, we still make use of our knowledge of the theoretical distribution of sample estimates to draw inferences about the population parameter.

Sampling distribution of the mean

Suppose we are interested in estimating the population mean; we could take many repeated samples of size n from the population, and estimate the mean in each sample. A histogram of the estimates of these means would show their distribution (Fig. 10.1); this is the **sampling distribution of the mean**. We can show that:

- If the sample size is reasonably large, the estimates of the mean follow a **Normal** distribution, whatever the distribution of the original data in the population (this comes from a theorem known as the *Central Limit Theorem*).
- If the sample size is small, the estimates of the mean follow a Normal distribution provided the data in the population follow a Normal distribution.
- The mean of the estimates is an **unbiased** estimate of the true mean in the population, i.e. the mean of the estimates equals the true population mean.
- The variability of the distribution is measured by the standard deviation of the estimates; this is known as the **standard error of the mean** (often denoted by SEM). If we know the population standard deviation (σ), then the standard error of the mean is given by:

$$SEM = \sigma / \sqrt{n}$$

When we only have one sample, as is customary, our best estimate of the population mean is the sample mean, and because we rarely know the standard deviation in the population, we estimate the standard error of the mean by:

$$SEM = s / \sqrt{n}$$

where s is the standard deviation of the observations in the sample (Topic 6). The SEM provides a measure of the precision of our estimate.

Interpreting standard errors

- A **large** standard error indicates that the estimate is *imprecise*.

- A **small** standard error indicates that the estimate is *precise*.

The standard error is reduced, i.e. we obtain a more precise estimate, if:
- the size of the sample is increased (Fig. 10.1);
- the data are less variable.

SD or SEM?

Although these two parameters seem to be similar, they are used for different purposes. The standard deviation describes the variation in the data values and should be quoted if you wish to illustrate variability in the data. In contrast, the standard error describes the precision of the sample mean, and should be quoted if you are interested in the mean of a set of data values.

Sampling distribution of a proportion

We may be interested in the proportion of individuals in a population who possess some characteristic. Having taken a sample of size n from the population, our best estimate, p, of the population proportion, π, is given by:

$$p = r/n$$

where r is the number of individuals in the sample with the characteristic. If we were to take repeated samples of size n from our population and plot the estimates of the proportion as a histogram, the resulting **sampling distribution of the proportion** would approximate a Normal distribution with mean value, π. The standard deviation of this distribution of estimated proportions is the **standard error of the proportion**. When we take only a single sample, it is estimated by:

$$SE(p) = \sqrt{\frac{p(1-p)}{n}}$$

This provides a measure of the precision of our estimate of π; a small standard error indicates a precise estimate.

Example

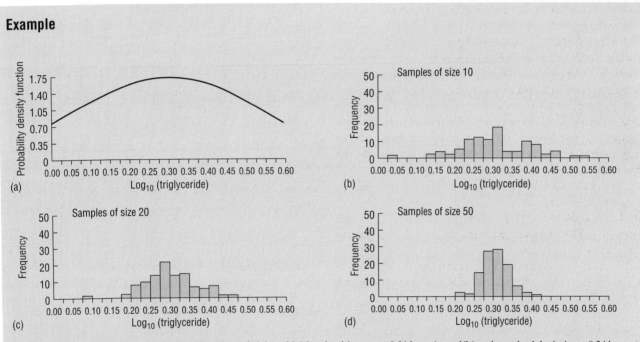

Fig. 10.1 (a) Theoretical Normal distribution of $\log_{10}$ (triglyceride) levels with mean = 0.31 $\log_{10}$ (mmol/L) and standard deviation = 0.24 $\log_{10}$ (mmol/L), and the observed distributions of the means of 100 random samples of size (b) 10, (c) 20, and (d) 50 taken from this theoretical distribution.

11 Confidence intervals

Once we have taken a sample from our population, we obtain a point estimate (Topic 10) of the parameter of interest, and calculate its standard error to indicate the precision of the estimate. However, to most people the standard error is not, by itself, particularly useful. It is more helpful to incorporate this measure of precision into an **interval estimate** for the population parameter. We do this by using our knowledge of the theoretical probability distribution of the sample statistic to calculate a **confidence interval** (**CI**) for the parameter. Generally, the confidence interval extends either side of the estimate by some multiple of the standard error; the two values (the **confidence limits**) defining the interval are generally separated by a comma and contained in brackets.

Confidence interval for the mean

Using the Normal distribution

The sample mean, $\bar{x}$, follows a Normal distribution if the sample size is large (Topic 10). Therefore we can make use of our knowledge of the Normal distribution when considering the sample mean. In particular, 95% of the distribution of sample means lies within 1.96 standard deviations (SD) of the population mean. When we have a single sample, we call this SD the standard error of the mean (SEM), and calculate the 95% **confidence interval for the mean** as:

$$(\bar{x} - (1.96 \times \text{SEM}), \bar{x} + (1.96 \times \text{SEM}))$$

If we were to repeat the experiment many times, the interval would contain the true population mean on 95% of occasions. We usually interpret this confidence interval as the range of values within which we are 95% confident that the true population mean lies. Although not strictly correct (the population mean is a fixed value and therefore cannot have a probability attached to it), we will interpret the confidence interval in this way as it is conceptually easier to understand.

Using the *t*-distribution

We can only use the Normal distribution if we know the value of the variance in the population. Furthermore if the sample size is small the sample mean only follows a Normal distribution if the underlying population data are Normally distributed. Where the underlying data are not Normally distributed, and/or we do not know the population variance, the sample mean follows a *t*-distribution (Topic 8). We calculate the 95% confidence interval for the mean as:

$$(\bar{x} - (t_{0.05} \times \text{SEM}), \bar{x} + (t_{0.05} \times \text{SEM}))$$

i.e. it is $\quad \bar{x} \pm t_{0.05} \times \dfrac{s}{\sqrt{n}}$

where $t_{0.05}$ is the **percentage point** (percentile) of the *t*-distribution (Appendix A2) with $(n - 1)$ degrees of freedom which gives a two-tailed probability (Topic 17) of 0.05. This generally provides a slightly wider confidence interval than that using the Normal distribution to allow for the extra uncertainty that we have introduced by estimating the population standard deviation and/or because of the small sample size. When the sample size is large, the difference between the two distributions is negligible. *Therefore, we always use the t-distribution when calculating confidence intervals even if the sample size is large.*

By convention we usually quote 95% confidence intervals. We could calculate other confidence intervals, e.g. a 99% CI for the mean. Instead of multiplying the standard error by the tabulated value of the *t*-distribution corresponding to a two-tailed probability of 0.05, we multiply it by that corresponding to a two-tailed probability of 0.01. This is wider than a 95% confidence interval, to reflect our increased confidence that the range includes the population mean.

Confidence interval for the proportion

The sampling distribution of a proportion follows a Binomial distribution (Topic 8). However, if the sample size, n, is reasonably large, then the sampling distribution of the proportion is approximately Normal with mean, π. We estimate π by the proportion in the sample, $p = r/n$ (where r is the number of individuals in the sample with the characteristic of interest), and its standard error is estimated by $\sqrt{\dfrac{p(1-p)}{n}}$ (Topic 10).

The 95% confidence interval for the proportion is estimated by:

$$\left(p - \left[1.96 \times \sqrt{\frac{p(1-p)}{n}} \right], \quad p + \left[1.96 \times \sqrt{\frac{p(1-p)}{n}} \right] \right)$$

If the sample size is small (usually when np or $n(1 - p)$ is less than 5) then we have to use the Binomial distribution to calculate exact confidence intervals[1]. Note that if p is expressed as a percentage, we replace $(1-p)$ by $(100-p)$.

Interpretation of confidence intervals

When interpreting a confidence interval we are interested in a number of issues.

[1] Ciba-Geigy Ltd. (1990) *Geigy Scientific Tables*, Vol. 2, 8th edn. Ciba-Geigy Ltd., Basle.

- **How wide is it?** A wide confidence interval indicates that the estimate is imprecise; a narrow one indicates a precise estimate. The width of the confidence interval depends on the size of the standard error, which in turn depends on the sample size and, when considering a numerical variable, the variability of the data. Therefore, small studies on variable data give wider confidence intervals than larger studies on less variable data.
- **What clinical implications can be derived from it?** The upper and lower limits provide a means of assessing whether the results are clinically important (see Example).
- **Does it include any values of particular interest?** We can check whether a hypothesized value for the population parameter falls within the confidence interval. If so, then our results are consistent with this hypothesized value. If not, then it is unlikely (for a 95% confidence interval, the chance is at most 5%) that the parameter has this value.

Degrees of freedom

You will come across the term 'degrees of freedom' in statistics. In general they can be calculated as the sample size minus the number of constraints in a particular calculation; these constraints may be the parameters that have to be estimated. As a simple illustration, consider a set of three numbers which add up to a particular total (T). Two of the numbers are 'free' to take any value but the remaining number is fixed by the single constraint imposed by T. Therefore the numbers have two degrees of freedom. Similarly, the degrees of freedom of the sample variance, $s^2 = \frac{\sum (x - \bar{x})^2}{n-1}$ (Topic 6), are the sample size minus one, because we have to calculate the sample mean ($\bar{x}$), an estimate of the population mean, in order to evaluate s^2.

Example

Confidence interval for the mean

We are interested in determining the mean age at first birth in women who have bleeding disorders. In a sample of 49 such women (Topic 2):

Mean age at birth of child, $\bar{x} = 27.01$ years
Standard deviation, $s = 5.1282$ years
Standard error, SEM $= \frac{5.1282}{\sqrt{49}} = 0.7326$ years

The variable is approximately Normally distributed but, because the population variance is unknown, we use the t-distribution to calculate the confidence interval. The 95% confidence interval for the mean is:

$$27.01 \pm (2.011 \times 0.7326) = (25.54, 28.48) \text{ years}$$

where 2.011 is the percentage point of the t-distribution with $(49 - 1) = 48$ degrees of freedom giving a two-tailed probability of 0.05 (Appendix A2).

We are 95% certain that the true mean age at first birth in women with bleeding disorders in the population ranges from 25.54 to 28.48 years. This range is fairly narrow, reflecting a precise estimate. In the general population, the mean age at first birth in 1997 was 26.8 years. As 26.8 falls into our confidence interval, there is little evidence that women with bleeding disorders tend to give birth at an older age than other women.

Note that the 99% confidence interval (25.05, 28.97 years), is slightly wider than the 95% CI, reflecting our increased confidence that the population mean lies in the interval.

Confidence interval for the proportion

Of the 64 women included in the study, 27 (42.2%) reported that they experienced bleeding gums at least once a week. This is a relatively high percentage, and may provide a way of identifying undiagnosed women with bleeding disorders in the general population. We calculate a 95% confidence interval for the proportion with bleeding gums in the population.

Sample proportion $= 27/64 = 0.422$
Standard error of proportion $= \sqrt{\frac{0.422(1-0.422)}{64}} = 0.0617$
95% confidence interval $= 0.422 \pm (1.96 \times 0.0617)$
$= (0.301, 0.543)$

We are 95% certain that the true percentage of women with bleeding disorders in the population who experience bleeding gums this frequently ranges from 30.1% to 54.3%. This is a fairly wide confidence interval, suggesting poor precision; a larger sample size would enable us to obtain a more precise estimate. However, the upper and lower limits of this confidence interval both indicate that a substantial percentage of these women are likely to experience bleeding gums. We would need to obtain an estimate of the frequency of this complaint in the general population before drawing any conclusions about its value for identifying undiagnosed women with bleeding disorders.

12 Study design I

Study design is vitally important as poorly designed studies may give misleading results. Large amounts of data from a poor study will not compensate for problems in its design. In this topic and in Topic 13 we discuss some of the main aspects of study design. In Topics 14–16 we discuss specific types of study: clinical trials, cohort studies and case–control studies.

The aims of any study should be clearly stated at the outset. We may wish to estimate a parameter in the population (such as the risk of some event), to consider associations between a particular aetiological factor and an outcome of interest, or to evaluate the effect of an intervention (such as a new treatment). There may be a number of possible designs for any such study. The ultimate choice of design will depend not only on the aims, but on the resources available and ethical considerations (see Table 12.1).

Experimental or observational studies

- **Experimental** studies involve the investigator intervening in some way to affect the outcome. The clinical trial (Topic 14) is an example of an experimental study in which the investigator introduces some form of treatment. Other examples include animal studies or laboratory studies that are carried out under experimental conditions. Experimental studies provide the most convincing evidence for any hypothesis as it is generally possible to control for factors that may affect the outcome. However, these studies are not always feasible or, if they involve humans or animals, may be unethical.
- **Observational** studies, for example cohort (Topic 15) or case–control (Topic 16) studies, are those in which the investigator does nothing to affect the outcome, but simply observes what happens. These studies may provide poorer information than experimental studies because it is often impossible to control for all factors that affect the outcome. However, in some situations, they may be the only types of study that are helpful or possible. **Epidemiological studies**, which assess the relationship between factors of interest and disease in the population, are observational.

Assessing causality in observational studies

Although the most convincing evidence for the causal role of a factor in disease usually comes from experimental studies, information from observational studies may be used provided it meets a number of criteria. The most well known criteria for assessing causation were proposed by Hill[1].

[1] Hill, A.B. (1965) The environment and disease: association or causation? *Proceedings of the Royal Society of Medicine*, **58**, 295.

- The cause must precede the effect.
- The association should be plausible, i.e. the results should be biologically sensible.
- There should be consistent results from a number of studies.
- The association between the cause and the effect should be strong.
- There should be a dose–response relationship with the effect, i.e. higher levels of the effect should lead to more severe disease or more rapid disease onset.
- Removing the factor of interest should reduce the risk of disease.

Cross-sectional or longitudinal studies

- **Cross-sectional** studies are carried out at a single point in time. Examples include surveys and censuses of the population. They are particularly suitable for estimating the **point prevalence** of a condition in the population.

$$\text{Point prevalence} = \frac{\text{Number with the disease at a single time point}}{\text{Total number studied at the same time point}}$$

As we do not know when the events occurred prior to the study, we can only say that there is an association between the factor of interest and disease, and not that the factor is likely to have *caused* disease. Furthermore, we cannot estimate the **incidence** of the disease, i.e. the rate of new events in a particular period. In addition, because cross-sectional studies are only carried out at one point in time, we cannot consider trends over time. However, these studies are generally quick and cheap to perform.

- **Longitudinal studies** follow a sample of individuals over time. They are usually **prospective** in that individuals are followed forwards from some point in time (Topic 15). Sometimes **retrospective** studies, in which individuals are selected and factors that have occurred in their past are identified (Topic 16), are also perceived as longitudinal. Longitudinal studies generally take longer to carry out than cross-sectional studies, thus requiring more resources, and, if they rely on patient memory or medical records, may be subject to bias (explained at the end of this topic).
- **Repeated cross-sectional** studies may be carried out at different time points to assess trends over time. However, as these studies involve different groups of individuals at each time point, it can be difficult to assess whether apparent changes over time simply reflect differences in the groups of individuals studied.

Experimental studies are generally prospective as they consider the impact of an intervention on an outcome that will happen in the future. However, observational studies may be either prospective or retrospective

Controls

The use of a comparison group, or **control group**, is essential when designing a study and interpreting any research findings. For example, when assessing the causal role of a particular factor for a disease, the risk of disease should be considered both in those who are exposed and in those who are unexposed to the factor of interest (Topics 15 and 16). See also 'Treatment comparisons' in Topic 14.

Bias

When there is a systematic difference between the results from a study and the true state of affairs, bias is said to have occurred. Types of bias include:

- **Observer bias**—one observer consistently under- or over-reports a particular variable;
- **Confounding bias**—where a spurious association arises due to a failure to adjust fully for factors related to both the risk factor and outcome;
- **Selection bias**—patients selected for inclusion into a study are not representative of the population to which the results will be applied;
- **Information bias**—measurements are incorrectly recorded in a systematic manner; and
- **Publication bias**—a tendency to publish only those papers that report positive or topical results.

Other biases may, for example, be due to **recall** (Topic 16), **healthy entrant effect** (Topic 15), **assessment** (Topic 14) and **allocation** (Topic 14).

Table 12.1 Study designs.

Type of study	Timing	Form	Action in past time	Action in present time (starting point)	Action in future time	Typical uses
Cross-sectional	Cross-sectional	Observational		Collect all information		• Prevalence estimates • Reference ranges and diagnostic tests • Current health status of a group
Repeated cross-sectional	Cross-sectional	Observational		Collect all information	Collect all information	Collect all information	• Changes over time
Cohort (Topic 15)	Longitudinal (prospective)	Observational		Define cohort and assess risk factors → follow → Observe outcomes		• Prognosis and natural history (what will happen to someone with disease) • Aetiology
Case-control (Topic 16)	Longitudinal (retrospective)	Observational	Assess risk factors	← trace ← Define cases and controls (i.e. outcome)		• Aetiology (particularly for rare diseases)
Experiment	Longitudinal (prospective)	Experimental		Apply intervention → follow → Observe outcomes		• Clinical trial to assess therapy (Topic 14) • Trial to assess preventative measure, e.g. large scale vaccine trial • Laboratory experiment

13 Study design II

Variation

Variation in data may be caused by known factors, measurement 'errors', or may be **unexplainable random variation**. We measure the impact of variation in the data on the estimation of a population parameter by using the standard error (Topic 10). When the measurement of a variable is subject to considerable variation, estimates relating to that variable will be imprecise, with large standard errors. Clearly, it is desirable to reduce the impact of variation as far as possible, and thereby increase the precision of our estimates. There are various ways in which we can do this.

Replication

Our estimates are more precise if we take replicates (e.g. two or three measurements of a given variable for every individual on each occasion). However, as replicate measurements are not independent, we must take care when analysing these data. A simple approach is to use the mean of each set of replicates in the analysis in place of the original measurements. Alternatively, we can use methods that specifically deal with replicated measurements.

Sample size

The choice of an appropriate size for a study is a crucial aspect of study design. With an increased sample size, the standard error of an estimate will be reduced, leading to increased precision and study power (Topic 18). Sample size calculations (Topic 33) should be carried out before starting the study.

Particular study designs

Modifications of simple study designs can lead to more precise estimates. Essentially we are comparing the effect of one or more '**treatments**' on **experimental units**. The experimental unit is the smallest group of 'individuals' who can be regarded as independent for the purposes of analysis, for example, an individual patient, volume of blood or skin patch. If experimental units are assigned randomly (i.e. by chance) to treatments (Topic 14) and there are no other refinements to the design, then we have a **complete randomized design**. Although this design is straightforward to analyse, it is inefficient if there is substantial variation between the experimental units. In this situation, we can incorporate **blocking** and/or use a **cross-over design** to reduce the impact of this variation.

Blocking

It is often possible to group experimental units that share similar characteristics into a homogeneous **block** or **stratum** (e.g. the blocks may represent different age groups). The variation between units in a block is less than that between units in different blocks. The individuals within each block are randomly assigned to treatments; we compare treatments within each block rather than making an overall comparison between the individuals in different blocks. We can therefore assess the effects of treatment more precisely than if there was no blocking.

Parallel versus cross-over designs (Fig. 13.1)

Generally, we make comparisons between individuals in different groups. For example, most clinical trials (Topic 14) are **parallel** trials, in which each patient receives one of the two (or occasionally more) treatments that are being compared, i.e. they result in *between-individual* comparisons.

Because there is usually less variation in a measurement within an individual than between different individuals (Topic 6), in some situations it may be preferable to consider using each individual as his/her own control. These *within-individual* comparisons provide more precise comparisons than those from between-individual designs, and fewer individuals are required for the study to achieve the same level of precision. In a clinical trial setting, the **cross-over** design[1] is an example of a within-individual comparison; if there are two treatments, every individual gets each treatment, one after the other in a random order to eliminate any effect of calendar time. The treatment periods are separated by a **washout period**, which allows any residual effects (**carry-over**) of the previous treatment to dissipate. We analyse the difference in the responses on the two treatments for each individual. This design can only be used when the treatment temporarily alleviates symptoms rather than provides a cure, and the response time is not prolonged.

Factorial experiments

When we are interested in more than one factor, separate studies that assess the effect of varying one factor at a time may be inefficient and costly. **Factorial designs** allow the simultaneous analysis of any number of **factors** of interest. The simplest design, a 2×2 factorial experiment, considers two factors (for example, two different treatments), each at two **levels** (e.g. either active or inactive treatment). As

[1] Senn, S. (1993) *Cross-over Trials in Clinical Research*. Wiley, Chichester.

an example, consider the US Physicians Health study[2], designed to assess the importance of aspirin and beta carotene in preventing heart disease. A 2 × 2 factorial design was used with the two factors being the different compounds and the two levels being whether or not the physician received each compound. Table 13.1 shows the possible treatment combinations.

We assess the effect of the level of beta carotene by comparing patients in the left-hand column to those in the right-hand column. Similarly, we assess the effect of the level of aspirin by comparing patients in the top row with those in the bottom row. In addition, we can test whether the two factors are **interactive**, i.e. when the effect of the level of beta carotene is different for the two levels of aspirin. We

[2] Steering Committee of the Physician's Health Study Research Group. (1989) Final report of the aspirin component of the on-going Physicians Health Study. *New England Journal of Medicine*, **321**, 129–135.

then say that there is an **interaction** between the two factors. In this example, an interaction would suggest that the combination of aspirin and beta carotene together is more (or less) effective than would be expected by simply adding the separate effects of each drug. This design, therefore, provides additional information to two separate studies and is a more efficient use of resources, requiring a smaller sample size to obtain estimates with a given degree of precision.

Table 13.1 Possible treatment combinations.

	Beta carotene	
Aspirin	No	Yes
No	Nothing	Beta carotene
Yes	Aspirin	Aspirin + beta carotene

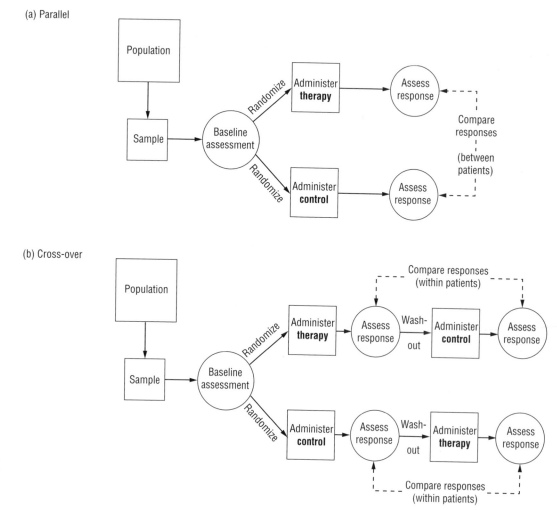

Fig. 13.1 (a) Parallel, and (b) cross-over designs.

14 Clinical trials

A **clinical trial**[1] is any form of planned experimental study designed, in general, to evaluate a new treatment on a clinical outcome in humans. Clinical trials may either be pre-clinical studies, small clinical studies to investigate effect and safety (**Phase I/II** trials), or full evaluations of the new treatment (**Phase III** trials). In this topic we discuss the main aspects of Phase III trials, all of which should be reported in any publication (see CONSORT statement, Table 14.1, and see Figs 14.1 & 14.2).

Treatment comparisons

Clinical trials are prospective studies, in that we are interested in measuring the impact of a treatment given now on a future possible outcome. In general, clinical trials evaluate a new intervention (e.g. type or dose of drug, or surgical procedure). Throughout this topic we assume, for simplicity, that a single new treatment is being evaluated.

An important feature of a clinical trial is that it should be comparative (Topic 12). Without a **control** treatment, it is impossible to be sure that any response is solely due to the effect of the treatment, and the importance of the new treatment can be over-stated. The control may be the standard treatment (a **positive control**) or, if one does not exist, may be a **negative control**, which can be a **placebo** (a treatment which looks and tastes like the new drug but which does not contain any active compound) or the absence of treatment if ethical considerations permit.

Endpoints

We must decide in advance which outcome most accurately reflects the benefit of the new therapy. This is known as the **primary endpoint** of the study and usually relates to treatment **efficacy**. **Secondary endpoints**, which often relate to toxicity, are of interest and should also be considered at the outset. Generally, all these endpoints are analysed at the end of the study. However, we may wish to carry out some preplanned **interim analyses** (for example, to ensure that no major toxicities have occurred requiring the trial to be stopped). Care should be taken when comparing treatments at these times due to the problems of multiple hypothesis testing (Topic 18).

Treatment allocation

Once a patient has been formally entered into a clinical trial, he/she is allocated to a treatment group. In general,

patients are allocated in a random manner (i.e. based on chance), using a process known as **random allocation** or **randomization**. This is often performed using a computer-generated list of random numbers or by using a table of random numbers (Appendix A12). For example, to allocate patients to two treatments, we might follow a sequence of random numbers, and allocate the patient to treatment A if the number is even and to treatment B if it is odd. This process promotes similarity between the treatment groups in terms of baseline characteristics at entry to the trial (i.e. it avoids **allocation bias**), maximizing the efficiency of the trial. Trials in which patients are randomized to receive either the new treatment or a control treatment are known as **randomized controlled trials** (often referred to as **RCTs**), and are regarded as optimal.

Further refinements of randomization, including **stratified randomization** (which controls for the effects of important factors), and **blocked randomization** (which ensures roughly equal sized treatment groups) exist. **Systematic allocation**, whereby patients are allocated to treatment groups systematically, possibly by day of visit, or date of birth, should be avoided where possible; the clinician may be able to determine the proposed treatment for a particular patient before he/she is entered into the trial, and this may influence his/her decision as to whether to include a patient in the trial. Sometimes we use a process known as **cluster randomization**, whereby we randomly allocate *groups* of individuals (e.g. all people registered at a single general practice) to treatments rather than each individual. We should take care when planning the size of the study and analysing the data in such designs[2].

Blinding

There may be **assessment bias** when patients and/or clinicians are aware of the treatment allocation, particularly if the response is subjective. An awareness of the treatment allocation may influence the recording of signs of improvement, or adverse events. Therefore, where possible, all participants (clinicians, patients, assessors) in a trial should be **blinded** to the treatment allocation. A trial in which both the patient and clinician/assessor are unaware of the treatment allocation is a **double-blind trial**. Trials in which it is impossible to blind the patient may be **single-blind** providing the clinician and/or assessor is blind to the treatment allocation.

[1] Pocock, S.J. (1983) *Clinical Trials: A Practical Approach*. Wiley, Chichester.

[2] Kerry, S.M. & Bland, J.M. (1998) Sample size in cluster randomisation. *British Medical Journal*, **316**, 549.

Patient issues

As clinical trials involve humans, patient issues are of importance. In particular, any clinical trial must be passed by an **ethical committee** who judge that the trial does not contravene the Declaration of Helsinki. **Informed patient consent** must be obtained from all patients before they are entered into a trial.

The protocol

Before any clinical trial is carried out, a written description of all aspects of the trial, known as the **protocol**, should be prepared. This includes information on the aims and objectives of the trial, along with a definition of which patients are to be recruited (**inclusion** and **exclusion criteria**), treatment schedules, data collection and analysis, contingency plans should problems arise, and study personnel. It is important to recruit enough patients into a trial so that the chance of correctly detecting a true treatment effect is sufficiently high. Therefore, before carrying out any clinical trial, the optimal **trial size** should be calculated (Topic 33).

Protocol deviations are patients who enter the trial but do not fulfil the protocol criteria, e.g. patients who were incorrectly recruited into or who withdrew from the study, and patients who switched treatments. To avoid bias, the study should be analysed on an **intention-to-treat** basis, in which all patients on whom we have information are analysed in the groups to which they were originally allocated, irrespective of whether they followed the treatment regime. Where possible, attempts should be made to collect information on patients who withdraw from the trial. **On-treatment** analyses, in which patients are only included in the analysis if they complete a *full* course of treatment, are not recommended as they often lead to biased treatment comparisons.

Table 14.1 A summary of the CONSORT (**Con**solidation of **S**tandards **for R**eporting **T**rials) statement's format for an optimally reported randomized controlled trial.

Heading	Descriptor
Title	*Identify* the study as a randomized trial
Abstract	*Use* a structured format
Introduction	*State* aims and specific objectives, and planned subgroup analyses
Methods	
Protocol	*Describe*:
	Planned study population, with inclusion/exclusion criteria
	Planned interventions (e.g. treatments) and their timing
	Primary and secondary outcome measure(s)
	Basis of sample size calculations (Topic 33)
	Rationale and methods for statistical analyses, and whether they were completed on an intention-to-treat basis
Assignment	*Describe*:
	Unit of randomization (e.g. individual, cluster)
	Method used to generate the randomization schedule
	Method of allocation concealment (e.g. sealed envelopes) and timing of assignment
Blinding	*Describe*:
	Similarity of treatments (e.g. appearance, taste of capsules/tablets)
	Mechanisms of blinding patients/clinicians/assessors
	Process of 'unblinding', if required
Results	
Particpant flow	*Provide* a trial profile (Fig. 14.1)
Analysis	*State* estimated effect of intervention on primary and secondary outcome measures, including a point estimate and measure of precision (confidence interval)
	State results in absolute numbers when feasible (e.g. 10/20 not just 50%)
	Present summary data and appropriate descriptive and inferential statistics
	Describe factors influencing response by treatment group, and any attempt to adjust for them
	Describe protocol deviations (with reasons)
Comment	*State* specific interpretation of study findings, including sources of bias and imprecision, and comparability with other studies
	State general interpretation of the data in light of all the available evidence

Adapted from: Begg, C., Cho, M., Eastwood, S., *et al.* (1996) Improving the quality of reporting of randomized controlled trials. The CONSORT statement. *Journal of the American Medical Association*, **276**, 637–639. (Copyrighted 1996, American Medical Association.)

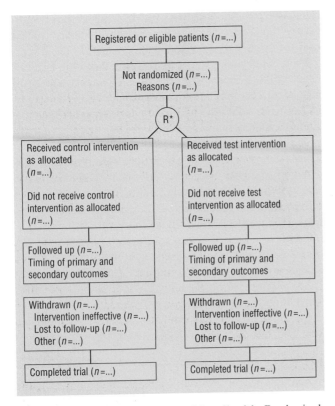

Fig. 14.1 The CONSORT statement's trial profile of the Randomized Controlled Trial's progress, adapted from Begg *et al.* (1996). (* The 'R' indicates randomization.) (Copyrighted 1996, American Medical Association.)

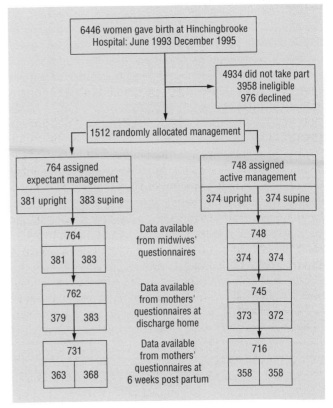

Fig. 14.2 Trial profile example (adapted from trial described in Topic 37 with permission).

5 Cohort studies

A cohort study takes a group of individuals and usually follows them forward in time, the aim being to study whether exposure to a particular aetiological factor will affect the incidence of a disease outcome in the future (Fig. 15.1). If so, the factor is known as a **risk factor** for the disease outcome. For example, a number of cohort studies have investigated the relationship between dietary factors and cancer. Although most cohort studies are prospective, **historical** cohorts can be investigated, the information being obtained retrospectively. However, the quality of historical studies is often dependent on medical records and memory, and they may therefore be subject to bias.

Cohort studies can either be fixed or dynamic. If individuals leave a **fixed** cohort, they are not replaced. In **dynamic** cohorts, individuals may drop out of the cohort, and new individuals may join as they become eligible.

Selection of cohort

The cohort should be representative of the population to which the results will be generalized. It is often advantageous if the individuals can be recruited from a similar source, such as a particular occupational group (e.g. civil servants, medical practitioners) as information on mortality and morbidity can be easily obtained from records held at the place of work, and individuals can be re-contacted when necessary. However, such a cohort may not be truly representative of the general population, and may be healthier. Cohorts can also be recruited from GP lists, ensuring that a group of individuals with different health states is included in the study. However, these patients tend to be of similar social backgrounds because they live in the same area.

When trying to assess the aetiological effect of a risk factor, individuals recruited to cohorts should be disease-free at the start of the study. This is to ensure that any exposure to the risk factor occurs before the outcome, thus enabling a causal role for the factor to be postulated. Because individuals are disease-free at the start of the study, we often see a **healthy entrant** effect. Mortality rates in the first period of the study are then often lower than would be expected in the general population. This will be apparent when mortality rates start to increase suddenly a few years into the study.

Follow-up of individuals

When following individuals over time, there is always the problem that they may be lost to **follow-up**. Individuals may move without leaving a forwarding address, or they may decide that they wish to leave the study. The benefits of cohort studies are reduced if a large number of individuals is lost to follow-up. We should thus find ways to minimize these drop-outs, e.g. by maintaining regular contact with the individuals.

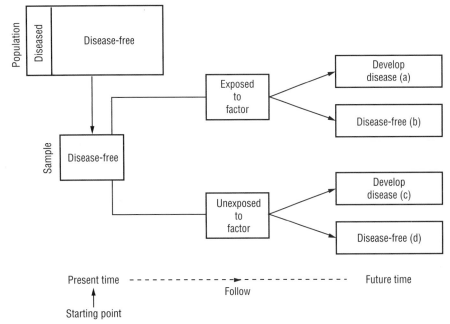

Fig. 15.1 Diagrammatic representation of a cohort study (frequencies in parenthesis, see Table 15.1).

Information on outcomes and exposures

It is important to obtain full and accurate information on disease outcomes, e.g. mortality and illness from different causes. This may entail searching through disease registries, mortality statistics, GP and hospital records.

Exposure to the risks of interest may change over the study period. For example, when assessing the relationship between alcohol consumption and heart disease, an individual's typical alcohol consumption is likely to change over time. Therefore it is important to re-interview individuals in the study on repeated occasions to study changes in exposure over time.

Analysis of cohort studies

Table 15.1 contains observed frequencies.

Table 15.1. Observed frequencies (see Fig. 15.1)

	Exposed to factor		
	Yes	No	Total
Disease of interest			
Yes	a	b	$a+b$
No	c	d	$c+d$
Total	$a+c$	$b+d$	$n=a+b+c+d$

Because patients are followed longitudinally over time, it is possible to estimate the **risk** of developing the disease in the population, by calculating the risk in the sample studied.

Estimated risk of disease

$$= \frac{\text{Number developing disease over study period}}{\text{Total number in the cohort}} = \frac{a+b}{n}$$

The risk of disease in the individuals exposed and unexposed to the factor of interest in the population can be estimated in the same way.

Estimated risk of disease in the exposed group,
$$\text{risk}_{\text{exp}} = a/(a+c)$$

Estimated risk of disease in the unexposed group,
$$\text{risk}_{\text{unexp}} = b/(b+d)$$

Then, **estimated relative risk** $= \dfrac{\text{risk}_{\text{exp}}}{\text{risk}_{\text{unexp}}}$

$$= \frac{a/(a+c)}{b/(b+d)}$$

The **relative risk** (RR) measures the increased (or decreased) risk of disease associated with exposure to the factor of interest. A relative risk of one indicates that the risk is the same in the exposed and unexposed groups. A relative risk greater than one indicates that there is an increased risk in the exposed group compared with the unexposed group; a relative risk less than one indicates a reduction in the risk of disease in the exposed group. For example, a relative risk of 2 would indicate that individuals in the exposed group had twice the risk of disease of those in the unexposed group.

Confidence intervals for the relative risk should be calculated, and we can test whether the relative risk is equal to one. These are easily performed on a computer and therefore we omit details.

Advantages of cohort studies

- The time sequence of events can be assessed.
- They can provide information on a wide range of outcomes.
- It is possible to measure the incidence/risk of disease directly.
- It is possible to collect very detailed information on exposure to a wide range of factors.
- It is possible to study exposure to factors that are rare.
- Exposure can be measured at a number of time points, so that changes in exposure over time can be studied.
- There is reduced **recall** and **selection bias** compared with case-control studies (Topic 16).

Disadvantages of cohort studies

- In general, cohort studies follow individuals for long periods of time, and are therefore costly to perform.
- Where the outcome of interest is rare, a very large sample size is needed.
- As follow-up increases, there is often increased loss of patients as they migrate or leave the study, leading to biased results.
- As a consequence of the long time-scale, it is often difficult to maintain consistency of measurements and outcomes over time. Furthermore, individuals may modify their behaviour after an initial interview.
- It is possible that disease outcomes and their probabilities, or the aetiology of disease itself, may change over time.

Example

The British Regional Heart Study is a large cohort study of 7735 men aged 40–59 years randomly selected from general practices in 24 British towns, with the aim of identifying risk factors for ischaemic heart disease. At recruitment to the study, the men were asked about a number of demographic and lifestyle factors, including information on cigarette smoking habits. Of the 7718 men who provided information on smoking status, 5899 (76.4%) had smoked at some stage during their lives (including those who were current smokers and those who were ex-smokers). Over the subsequent 10 years, 650 of these 7718 men (8.4%) had a myocardial infarction (MI). The results, displayed in the table, show the number (and percentage) of smokers and non-smokers who developed and did not develop a MI over the 10 year period.

	MI in subsequent 10 years		
Smoking status at baseline	Yes	No	Total
Ever smoked	563 (9.5%)	5336 (90.5%)	5899
Never smoked	87 (4.8%)	1732 (95.2%)	1819
Total	650 (8.4%)	7068 (71.6%)	7718

The estimated relative risk $= \dfrac{(563/5899)}{(87/1819)} = 2.00$.

It can be shown that the 95% confidence interval for the true relative risk is (1.60, 2.49).

We can interpret the relative risk to mean that a middle-aged man who has *ever* smoked is twice as likely to suffer a MI over the next 10 year period as a man who has *never* smoked. Alternatively, the risk of suffering a MI for a man who has ever smoked is 100% greater than that of a man who has never smoked.

Data kindly provided by Ms F.C. Lampe, Ms M. Walker and Dr P. Whincup, Department of Primary Care and Population Sciences, Royal Free and University College Medical School, Royal Free Campus, London, UK.

16 Case–control studies

A case–control study compares the characteristics of a group of patients with a particular disease outcome (the **cases**) to a group of individuals without a disease outcome (the **controls**), to see whether any factors occurred more or less frequently in the cases than the controls (Fig. 16.1). Such retrospective studies do not provide information on the prevalence or incidence of disease but may give clues as to which factors elevate or reduce the risk of disease.

Selection of cases

It is important to define whether **incident** cases (patients who are recruited at the time of diagnosis) or **prevalent** cases (patients who were already diagnosed before entering the study) should be recruited. Prevalent cases may have had time to reflect on their history of exposure to risk factors, especially if the disease is a well-publicized one such as cancer, and may have altered their behaviour after diagnosis. It is important to identify as many cases as possible so that the results carry more weight and the conclusions can be generalized to future populations. To this end, it may be necessary to access hospital lists and disease registries, and to include cases who died during the time period when cases and controls were defined, because their exclusion may lead to a biased sample of cases.

Selection of controls

Controls should be screened at entry to the study to ensure that they do not have the disease of interest. Sometimes there may be more than one control for each case. Where possible, controls should be selected from the same source as cases. Controls are often selected from hospitals. However, as risk factors related to one disease outcome may also be related to other disease outcomes, the selection of hospital-based controls may over-select individuals who have been exposed to the risk factor of interest, and may, therefore, not always be appropriate. It is often acceptable to select controls from the general population, although they may not be as motivated to take part in such a study, and response rates may therefore be poorer in controls than cases. The use of neighbourhood controls may ensure that cases and controls are from similar social backgrounds.

Matching

Many case–control studies are **matched** in order to select cases and controls who are as similar as possible. In general, it is useful to sex-match individuals (i.e. if the case is male, the control should also be male), and, sometimes, patients will be age-matched. However, it is important not to match on the basis of the risk factor of interest, or on any factor that falls within the causal pathway of the disease, as this will remove the ability of the study to assess any relationship between the risk factor and the disease. Unfortunately, matching does mean that the effect on disease of the variables that have been used for matching cannot be studied.

Analysis of unmatched case–control studies

Table 16.1 shows observed frequencies. Because patients are selected on the basis of their disease status, it is not possible to estimate the absolute risk of disease. We can calculate the **odds ratio**, which is given by:

$$\text{Odds ratio} = \frac{\text{Odds of being a case in the exposed group}}{\text{Odds of being a case in the unexposed group}}$$

Table 16.1 Observed frequencies (see Fig. 16.1).

	Exposed to factor		
	Yes	No	Total
Disease status			
Case	a	b	$a+b$
Control	c	d	$c+d$
Total	$a+c$	$b+d$	$n=a+b+c+d$

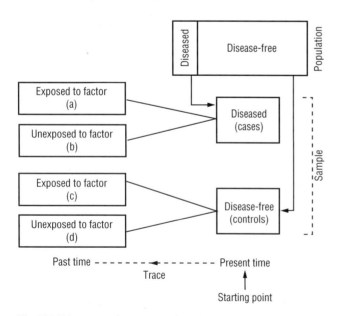

Fig. 16.1 Diagrammatic representation of a case–control study.

where, for example, the odds of being a case in the exposed group is equal to

$$\frac{\text{probability of being a case in the exposed group}}{\text{probability of not being a case in the exposed group}}$$

The odds of being a case in the exposed and unexposed samples are:

$$\text{odds}_{exp} = \frac{\left(\dfrac{a}{a+c}\right)}{\left(\dfrac{c}{a+c}\right)} = \frac{a}{c} \quad \text{odds}_{unexp} = \frac{\left(\dfrac{b}{b+d}\right)}{\left(\dfrac{d}{b+d}\right)} = \frac{b}{d}$$

and therefore the **estimated odds ratio** $= \dfrac{a/c}{b/d} = \dfrac{a \times d}{b \times c}$

When the incidence of disease is rare, the odds ratio is an estimate of the relative risk, and is interpreted in a similar way, i.e. it indicates the increased (or decreased) risk associated with exposure to the factor of interest. An odds ratio of one indicates that there is the same risk in the exposed and unexposed groups; an odds ratio greater than one indicates that there is an increased risk in the exposed group compared with the unexposed group, etc. Confidence intervals and hypothesis tests can also be generated for the odds ratio.

Analysis of matched case–control studies

Where possible, the analysis of matched case–control studies should allow for the fact that cases and controls are linked to each other as a result of the matching. Further details of methods of analysis for matched studies can be found in Breslow and Day[1].

Advantages of case–control studies

- They are generally relatively quick, cheap and easy to perform.
- They are particularly suitable for rare diseases.
- A wide range of risk factors can be investigated.
- There is no loss to follow-up.

Disadvantages of case–control studies

- **Recall bias**, when cases have a differential ability to remember certain details about their histories, is a potential problem. For example, a lung cancer patient may well remember the occasional period when he/she smoked, whereas a control may not remember a similar period.
- If the onset of disease preceded exposure to the risk factor, causation cannot be inferred.
- Case–control studies are not suitable when exposures to the risk factor are rare.

Example

A total of 1327 women aged 50–81 years with hip fractures, who lived in a largely urban area in Sweden, were investigated in this unmatched case–control study. They were compared with 3262 controls within the same age range randomly selected from the national register. Interest was centred on determining whether postmenopausal hormone replacement therapy (HRT) substantially reduced the risk of hip fracture. The results in the table show the number of women who were current users of HRT and those who had never used or formerly used HRT in the case and control groups.

The observed odds ratio $= (40 \times 3023)/(239 \times 1287)$
$= 0.39.$

It can be shown that the 95% confidence interval for the odds ratio is (0.28, 0.56).

	Current user of HRT	Never used HRT/former user of HRT	Total
With hip fracture (cases)	40 (14%)	1287 (30%)	1327
Without hip fracture (controls)	239	3023	3262
Total	279	4310	4589

A postmenopausal woman in this age range in Sweden who was a current user of HRT thus had 39% of the risk of a hip fracture of a woman who had never used or formerly used HRT, i.e. being a current user of HRT reduced the risk of hip fracture by 61%.

Data extracted from: Michaelsson, K., Baron, J.A., Farahmand, B.Y., *et al.* (1998) Hormone replacement therapy and risk of hip fracture: population based case–control study. *British Medical Journal,* **316,** 1858–1863.

[1] Breslow, N.E. & Day, N.E. (1980) *Statistical Methods in Cancer Research. Volume I — The Analysis of Case–control Studies.* International Agency for Cancer Research, Lyon.

17 Hypothesis testing

We often gather sample data in order to assess how much evidence there is against a specific hypothesis about the population. We use a process known as **hypothesis testing** (or **significance testing**) to quantify our belief against a particular hypothesis.

This topic describes the format of hypothesis testing in general (Box 17.1); details of specific hypothesis tests are given in subsequent topics. For easy reference, each hypothesis test is contained in a similarly formatted box.

Box 17.1 Hypothesis testing—a general overview
We define five stages when carrying out a hypothesis test:

1 Define the *null* and *alternative hypotheses* under study

2 Collect relevant data from a sample of individuals

3 Calculate the value of the *test-statistic* specific to H_0

4 Compare the value of the test statistic to values from a known probability distribution

5 Interpret the *P-value* and results

Defining the null and alternative hypotheses

We always test the **null hypothesis** (H_0), which assumes *no effect* (e.g. the difference in means equals zero) in the *population*. For example, if we are interested in comparing smoking rates in men and women in the population, the null hypothesis would be:

H_0: smoking rates are the same in men and women in the population

We then define the **alternative hypothesis** (H_1), which holds if the null hypothesis is not true. The alternative hypothesis relates more directly to the theory we wish to investigate. So, in the example, we might have:

H_1: the smoking rates are different in men and women in the population.

We have not specified any direction for the difference in smoking rates, i.e. we have not stated whether men have higher or lower rates than women in the population. This leads to what is known as a **two-tailed test**, because we allow for either eventuality, and is recommended as we are rarely certain, *in advance*, of the direction of any difference, if one exists. In some, very rare, circumstances, we may carry

out a **one-tailed test** in which a direction of effect is specified in H_1. This might apply if we are considering a disease from which all untreated individuals die; a new drug cannot make things worse.

Obtaining the test statistic

After collecting the data, we substitute values from our sample into a formula, specific to the test we are using, to determine a value for the **test statistic**. This reflects the amount of evidence in the data *against* the null hypothesis—usually, the larger the value, ignoring its sign, the greater the evidence.

Obtaining the *P*-value

All test statistics follow known theoretical probability distributions (Topics 7 and 8). We relate the value of the test statistic obtained from the sample to the known distribution to obtain the **P-value**, the area in both (or occasionally one) tails of the probability distribution. Most computer packages provide the two-tailed *P*-value automatically. **The P-value is the probability of obtaining our results, or something more extreme, if the null hypothesis is true.** The null hypothesis relates to the population of interest, rather than the sample. Therefore, the null hypothesis is either true or false and we *cannot* interpret the *P*-value as the probability that the null hypothesis is true.

Using the *P*-value

We must make a decision about how much evidence we require to enable us to decide to reject the null hypothesis in favour of the alternative. The smaller the *P*-value, the greater the evidence against the null hypothesis.

• Conventionally, we consider that if the *P*-value is less than 0.05, there is sufficient evidence to reject the null hypothesis, as there is only a small chance of the results occurring if the null hypothesis were true. We then *reject* the null hypothesis and say that the results are **significant** at the 5% level (Fig. 17.1).

• In contrast, if the *P*-value is greater than 0.05, we usually conclude that there is insufficient evidence to reject the null hypothesis. We *do not reject* the null hypothesis, and we say that the results are **not significant** at the 5% level (Fig. 17.1). This does not mean that the null hypothesis is true; simply that we do not have enough evidence to reject it.

The choice of 5% is arbitrary. On 5% of occasions we will incorrectly reject the null hypothesis when it is true. In situations in which the clinical implications of incorrectly rejecting the null hypothesis are severe, we may require stronger evidence before rejecting the null hypothesis (e.g.

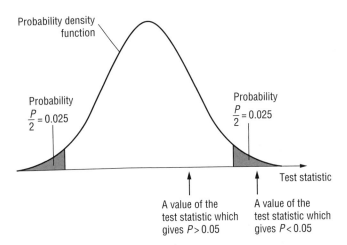

Probability density function

Probability $\frac{P}{2} = 0.025$

Probability $\frac{P}{2} = 0.025$

Test statistic

A value of the test statistic which gives $P > 0.05$

A value of the test statistic which gives $P < 0.05$

Fig. 17.1 Probability distribution of the test statistic showing a two-tailed probability, $P = 0.05$.

we may choose a P-value of 0.01, or 0.001). The chosen cut-off (e.g. 0.05 or 0.01) is called the **significance level** of the test.

Quoting a result only as significant at a certain cut-off level (e.g. 0.05) can be misleading. For example, if $P = 0.04$ we would reject H_0; however, if $P = 0.06$ we would not reject it. Are these really different? Therefore, we recommend quoting the exact P-value, often obtained from the computer output.

Non-parametric tests

Hypothesis tests which are based on knowledge of the probability distributions that the data follow are known as **parametric tests.** Often data do not conform to the assumptions that underly these methods (Topic 32). In these instances we can use **non-parametric tests** (sometimes referred to as **distribution-free** tests, or **rank methods**).

These tests generally replace the data with their ranks (i.e. the numbers 1, 2, 3 etc., describing their position in the ordered data set) and make no assumptions about the probability distribution that the data follow.

Non-parametric tests are particularly useful when the sample size is small (so that it is impossible to assess the distribution of the data), and when the data are measured on a categorical scale. However, non-parametric tests are generally wasteful of information; consequently they have less power (Topic 18) of detecting a real effect than the equivalent parametric test if all the assumptions underlying the parametric test are satisfied. Furthermore, they are primarily significance tests that often do not provide estimates of the effects of interest; they lead to decisions rather than an appreciation or understanding of the data.

Which test?

Deciding which statistical test to use depends on the design of the study, the type of variable and the distribution that the data being studied follow. The flow chart on the inside front cover will aid your decision.

Hypothesis tests versus confidence intervals

Confidence intervals (Topic 11) and hypothesis tests are closely linked. The primary aim of a hypothesis test is to make a decision and provide an exact P-value. Confidence intervals quantify the effect of interest (e.g. the difference in means), and enable us to assess the clinical implications of the results. However, because they provide a range of plausible values for the true effect, they can also be used to make a decision although exact P-values are not provided. For example, if the hypothesized value for the effect (e.g. zero) lies outside the 95% confidence interval then we believe the hypothesized value is implausible and would reject H_0. In this instance we know that the P-value is less than 0.05 but do not know its exact value.

18 Errors in hypothesis testing

Making a decision

Most hypothesis tests in medical statistics compare groups of people who are exposed to a variety of experiences. We may, for example, be interested in comparing the effectiveness of two forms of treatment for reducing 5 year mortality from breast cancer. For a given outcome (e.g. death), we call the *comparison of interest* (e.g. the difference in 5 year mortality rates) the **effect** of interest or, if relevant, the **treatment effect**. We express the null hypothesis in terms of no effect (e.g. the 5 year mortality from breast cancer is the same in two treatment groups); the two-sided alternative hypothesis is that the effect is not zero. We perform a hypothesis test that enables us to decide whether we have enough evidence to reject the null hypothesis (Topic 17). We can make one of two decisions; either we reject the null hypothesis, or we do not reject it.

Making the wrong decision

Although we hope we will draw the correct conclusion about the null hypothesis, we have to recognize that, because we only have a sample of information, we may make the wrong decision when we reject/do not reject the null hypothesis. The possible mistakes we can make are shown in Table 18.1.

- **Type I error**: *we reject the null hypothesis when it is true*, and conclude that there is an effect when, in reality, there is none. The maximum chance (probability) of making a Type I error is denoted by α (alpha). This is the significance level of the test (Topic 17); we reject the null hypothesis if our P-value is less than the significance level, i.e. if $P < \alpha$.

We must decide on the value of α before we collect our data; we usually assign a conventional value of 0.05 to it, although we might choose a more restrictive value such as 0.01. Our chance of making a Type I error will never exceed our chosen significance level, say $\alpha = 0.05$, because we will only reject the null hypothesis if $P < 0.05$. If we find that $P > 0.05$, we will not reject the null hypothesis, and, consequently, do not make a Type I error.

- **Type II error**: *we do not reject the null hypothesis when it is false*, and conclude that there is no effect when one really exists. The chance of making a Type II error is denoted by β (beta); its compliment, $(1 - \beta)$, is the **power** of the test. The power, therefore, is the *probability of rejecting the null hypothesis when it is false*; i.e. it is the chance (usually expressed as a percentage) of detecting, as statistically significant, a real treatment effect of a given size.

Ideally, we should like the power of our test to be 100%; we must recognize, however, that this is impossible because there is always a chance, albeit slim, that we could make a Type II error. Fortunately, however, we know which factors affect power, and thus we can control the power of a test by giving consideration to them.

Power and related factors

It is essential that we know the power of a proposed test at the planning stage of our investigation. Clearly, we should only embark on a study if we believe that it has a 'good' chance of detecting a clinically relevant effect, if one exists (by 'good' we mean that the power should be at least 70–80%). It is ethically irresponsible, and wasteful of time and resources, to undertake a clinical trial that has, say, only a 40% chance of detecting a real treatment effect.

A number of factors have a direct bearing on power for a given test.

- The **sample size**: power increases with increasing sample size. This means that a large sample has a greater ability than a small sample to detect a clinically important effect if it exists. When the sample size is very small, the test may have an inadequate power to detect a particular effect. We explain how to choose sample size, with power considerations, in Topic 33. The methods can also be used to evaluate the power of the test for a specified sample size.
- The **variability of the observations**: power increases as the variability of the observations decreases (Fig. 18.1).
- The **effect of interest**: the power of the test is greater for larger effects. A hypothesis test thus has a greater chance of detecting a large real effect than a small one.
- The **significance level**: the power is greater if the significance level is larger (this is equivalent to the probability of the Type I error (α) increasing as the probability of the Type II error (β) decreases). So, we are more likely to detect a real effect if we decide at the planning stage that we will regard our P-value as significant if it is less than 0.05 rather than less than 0.01. We can see this relationship between power and the significance level in Fig. 18.2.

Note that an inspection of the confidence interval (Topic 11) for the effect of interest gives an indication of whether the power of the test was adequate. A wide confidence interval results from a small sample and/or data with substantial variability, and is a suggestion of poor power.

Table 18.1 The consequences of hypothesis testing.

	Reject H_0	Do not reject H_0
H_0 true	Type I error	No error
H_0 false	No error	Type II error

Multiple hypothesis testing

Often, we want to carry out a number of significance tests on a data set, e.g. when it comprises many variables or there are more than two treatments. The Type I error rate increases dramatically as the number of comparisons increases, leading to spurious conclusions. Therefore, we should only perform a small number of tests, chosen to relate to the primary aims of the study and specified *a priori*. It is possible to use some form of *post-hoc* adjustment to the *P*-value to take account of the number of tests performed (Topic 22). For example, the **Bonferroni** approach (often regarded as rather conservative) multiplies each *P*-value by the number of tests carried out; any decisions about significance are then based on this adjusted *P*-value.

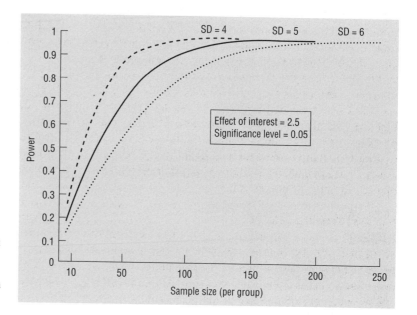

Fig. 18.1 Power curves showing the relationship between power and the sample size in each of two groups for the comparison of two means using the unpaired *t*-test. Each power curve relates to a two-sided test for which the significance level is 0.05, and the effect of interest (e.g. the difference between the treatment means) is 2.5. The assumed equal standard deviation of the measurements in the two groups is different for each power curve (see Example, Topic 33).

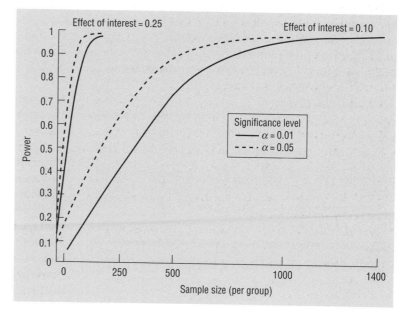

Fig. 18.2 Power curves showing the relationship between power and the sample size in each of two groups for the comparison of two proportions using the Chi-squared test. Curves are drawn when the effect of interest (e.g. the difference in the proportions with the characteristic of interest in the two treatment groups) is either 0.25 (i.e. 0.65–0.40) or 0.10 (i.e. 0.50–0.40); the significance level of the two-sided test is either 0.05 or 0.01 (see Example, Topic 33).

19 Numerical data: a single group

The problem

We have a sample from a single group of individuals and one numerical or ordinal variable of interest. We are interested in whether the average of this variable takes a particular value. For example, we may have a sample of patients with a specific medical condition. We have been monitoring triglyceride levels in the blood of healthy individuals and know that they have a geometric mean of 1.74 mmol/L. We wish to know whether the average level in our patients is the same as this value.

The one-sample *t*-test

Assumptions

In the population, the variable is Normally distributed with a given (usually unknown) variance. In addition, we have taken a reasonable sample size so that we can check the assumption of Normality (Topic 32).

Rationale

We are interested in whether the mean, μ, of the variable in the population of interest differs from some hypothesized value, μ_1. We use a test statistic that is based on the difference between the sample mean, $\bar{x}$, and μ_1. Assuming that we do not know the population variance, then this test statistic, often referred to as t, follows the t-distribution. If we do know the population variance, or the sample size is very large, then an alternative test (often called a z-test), based on the Normal distribution, may be used. However, in these situations, results from either test are virtually identical.

Additional notation

Our sample is of size n and the estimated standard deviation is s.

---

1 Define the null and alternative hypotheses under study

H_0: the mean in the population, μ, equals μ_1
H_1: the mean in the population does not equal μ_1.

2 Collect relevant data from a sample of individuals

3 Calculate the value of the test statistic specific to H_0

$$t = \frac{(\bar{x} - \mu_1)}{s/\sqrt{n}}$$

which follows the t-distribution with $(n-1)$ degrees of freedom.

continued

---

4 Compare the value of the test statistic to values from a known probability distribution

Refer t to Appendix A2.

5 Interpret the *P*-value and results

Interpret the P-value and calculate a confidence interval for the true mean in the population (Topic 11).

The 95% confidence interval is given by:

$$\bar{x} \pm t_{0.05} \times \left(s/\sqrt{n} \right)$$

where $t_{0.05}$ is the percentage point of the t-distribution with $(n-1)$ degrees of freedom which gives a two-tailed probability of 0.05.

Interpretation of the confidence interval

The 95% confidence interval provides a range of values in which we are 95% certain that the true population mean lies. If the 95% confidence interval does not include the hypothesized value for the mean, μ_1, we reject the null hypothesis at the 5% level. If, however, the confidence interval includes μ_1, then we fail to reject the null hypothesis at that level.

If the assumptions are not satisfied

We may be concerned that the variable does not follow a Normal distribution in the population. Whereas the t-test is relatively **robust** (Topic 32) to some degree of non-Normality, extreme skewness may be a concern. We can either transform the data, so that the variable is Normally distributed (Topic 9), or use a non-parametric test such as the sign test or Wilcoxon signed ranks test (Topic 20).

The sign test

Rationale

The sign test is a simple test based on the median of the distribution. We have some hypothesized value, λ, for the median in the population. If our sample comes from this population, then approximately half of the values in our sample should be greater than λ and half should be less than λ (after excluding any values which equal λ). The sign test considers the number of values in our sample that are greater (or less) than λ.

The sign test is a simple test; we can use a more powerful test, the Wilcoxon signed ranks test (Topic 20), which takes into account the ranks of the data as well as their signs when carrying out such an analysis.

---

1 Define the null and alternative hypotheses under study
H_0: the median in the population equals λ
H_1: the median in the population does not equal λ.

2 Collect relevant data from a sample of individuals

3 Calculate the value of the test statistic specific to H_0
Ignore all values that are equal to λ, leaving n' values. Count the values that are greater than λ. Similarly, count the values that are less than λ. (In practice this will often involve calculating the difference between each value in the sample and λ, and noting its sign.) Consider r, the smaller of these two counts.

- If $n' \leq 10$, the test statistic is r

- If $n' > 10$, calculate $z = \dfrac{\left| r - \dfrac{n'}{2} \right| - \dfrac{1}{2}}{\dfrac{\sqrt{n'}}{2}}$

where $n'/2$ is the number of values above (or below) the median that we would expect if the null hypothesis were true. The vertical bars indicate that we take the absolute (i.e. the positive) value of the number inside the bars. The distribution of z is approximately Normal. The subtraction of $1/2$ in the formula for z is a **continuity correction**, which we have to include to allow for the fact that we are relating a discrete value (r) to a continuous distribution (the Normal distribution).

4 Compare the value of the test statistic to values from a known probability distribution
- If $n' \leq 10$, refer r to Appendix A6
- If $n' > 10$, refer z to Appendix A1.

5 Interpret the P-value and results
Interpret the P-value and calculate a confidence interval for the median — some statistical packages provide this automatically; if not, we can rank the values in order of size and refer to Appendix A7 to identify the ranks of the values that are to be used to define the limits of the confidence interval. In general, confidence intervals for the median will be larger than those for the mean.

Example

There is some evidence that high blood triglyceride levels are associated with heart disease. As part of a large cohort study on heart disease, triglyceride levels were available in 232 men who developed heart disease over the 5 years after recruitment. We are interested in whether the average triglyceride levels in the population of men from which this sample is chosen is the same as that in the general population. A **one-sample t-test** was performed to investigate this. Triglyceride levels are skewed to the right (Fig. 8.3a); log triglyceride levels are approximately Normally distributed (Fig. 8.3b), so we performed our analysis on the log values. In the men in the general population, the mean of the log values equals $0.24 \log_{10}$ (mmol/L) equivalent to a geometric mean of 1.74 mmol/L.

---

1 H_0: the mean $\log_{10}$ (triglyceride level) in the population of men who develop heart disease equals $0.24 \log$ (mmol/L)

H_1: the mean $\log_{10}$ (triglyceride level) in the population of men who develop heart disease does not equal $0.24 \log$ (mmol/L)

2 Sample size, $n = 232$; mean of log values, $\bar{x} = 0.31 \log$ (mmol/L); standard deviation of log values, $s = 0.23 \log$ (mmol/L)

3 Test statistic, $t = \dfrac{0.31 - 0.24}{0.23 / \sqrt{232}} = 4.64$

4 We refer t to Appendix A2 with 231 degrees of freedom: $P < 0.001$

5 There is strong evidence to reject the null hypothesis that the geometric mean triglyceride level in the population of men who develop heart disease equals 1.74 mmol/L. The geometric mean triglyceride level in the population of men who develop heart disease is estimated as antilog $(0.31) = 10^{0.31}$, which equals 2.04 mmol/L. The 95% confidence interval for the geometric mean triglyceride level ranges from 1.90 to 2.19 mmol/l (i.e. antilog $[0.31 \pm 1.96 \times 0.23/\sqrt{232}]$). Therefore, in this population of patients, the geometric mean triglyceride level is significantly higher than that in the general population.

continued

We can use the **sign test** to carry out a similar analysis on the untransformed triglyceride levels as this does not make any distributional assumptions. We assume that the median and geometric mean triglyceride level in the male population are similar.

---

1 H_0: the median triglyceride level in the population of men who develop heart disease equals 1.74 mmol/L.

H_1: the median triglyceride level in the population of men who develop heart disease does not equal 1.74 mmol/L.

2 In this data set, the median value equals 1.94 mmol/L.

3 We investigate the differences between each value and 1.74. There are 231 non-zero differences, of which 134 are positive and 96 are negative. Therefore, $r = 96$. As the number of non-zero differences is greater than 10, we calculate:

$$z = \frac{\left| 96 - \frac{231}{2} \right| - \frac{1}{2}}{\sqrt{\frac{231}{2}}} = 2.50$$

4 We refer z to Appendix A1: $P = 0.012$.

5 There is evidence to reject the null hypothesis that the median triglyceride level in the population of men who develop heart disease equals 1.74 mmol/L. The formula in Appendix A7 indicates that the 95% confidence interval for the population median is given by the 101st and 132nd ranked values; these are 1.77 and 2.16 mmol/L. Therefore, in this population of patients, the median triglyceride level is significantly higher than that in the general population.

Data kindly provided by Ms F.C. Lampe, Ms M. Walker and Dr P. Whincup, Department of Primary Care and Population Sciences, Royal Free and University College Medical School, Royal Free Campus, London, UK.

20 Numerical data: two related groups

The problem

We have two samples that are related to each other and one numerical or ordinal variable of interest.

- The variable may be measured on each individual in two circumstances. For example, in a cross-over trial (Topic 13), each patient has two measurements on the variable, one while taking active treatment and one while taking placebo.
- The individuals in each sample may be different, but are linked to each other in some way. For example, patients in one group may be individually matched to patients in the other group in a case–control study (Topic 16).

Such data are known as **paired** data. It is important to take account of the dependence between the two samples when analysing the data, otherwise the advantages of pairing (Topic 13) are lost. We do this by considering the **differences** in the values for each pair, thereby reducing our two samples to a single sample of differences.

The paired *t*-test
Assumptions

In the population of interest, the individual differences are Normally distributed with a given (usually unknown) variance. We have a reasonable sample size so that we can check the assumption of Normality.

Rationale

If the two sets of measurements were the same, then we would expect the mean of the differences between each pair of measurements to be zero in the population of interest. Therefore, our test statistic simplifies to a one-sample *t*-test (Topic 19) on the differences, where the hypothesized value for the mean difference in the population is zero.

Additional notation

Because of the paired nature of the data, our two samples must be of the same size, n. We have n differences, with sample mean, $\bar{d}$, and estimated standard deviation s_d.

---

1 Define the null and alternative hypotheses under study

H_0: the mean difference in the population equals zero
H_1: the mean difference in the population does not equal zero.

continued

---

2 Collect relevant data from two related samples

3 Calculate the value of the test statistic specific to H_0

$$t = \frac{(\bar{d} - 0)}{\mathrm{SE}(\bar{d})} = \frac{\bar{d}}{s_d / \sqrt{n}}$$

which follows the *t*-distribution with $(n-1)$ degrees of freedom.

4 Compare the value of the test statistic to values from a known probability distribution

Refer t to Appendix A2.

5 Interpret the *P*-value and results

Interpret the *P*-value and calculate a confidence interval for the true mean difference in the population. The 95% confidence interval is given by

$$\bar{d} \pm t_{0.05} \times (s_d / \sqrt{n})$$

where $t_{0.05}$ is the percentage point of the *t*-distribution with $(n-1)$ degrees of freedom which gives a two-tailed probability of 0.05.

If the assumptions are not satisfied

If the differences do not follow a Normal distribution, the assumption underlying the *t*-test is not satisfied. We can either transform the data (Topic 9), or use a non-parametric test such as the sign test (Topic 19) or Wilcoxon signed ranks test to assess whether the differences are centred around zero.

The Wilcoxon signed ranks test
Rationale

In Topic 19, we explained how to use the **sign test** on a single sample of numerical measurements to test the null hypothesis that the population median equals a particular value. We can also use the sign test when we have **paired** observations, the pair representing matched individuals (e.g. in a case–control study, Topic 16) or measurements made on the same individual in different circumstances (as in a cross-over trial of two treatments, A and B, Topic 13). For each pair, we evaluate the **difference** in the measurements. The sign test can be used to assess whether the median difference in the population equals zero by considering the differences in the sample and observing how many are greater (or

49

less) than zero. However, the sign test does not incorporate information on the sizes of these differences.

The **Wilcoxon signed ranks test** takes account not only of the signs of the differences, but also their magnitude, and therefore is a more powerful test (Topic 18). The individual difference is calculated for each pair of results. Ignoring zero differences, these are then classed as being either positive or negative. In addition, the differences are placed in order of size, ignoring their signs, and are **ranked** accordingly. The smallest difference thus gets the value 1, the second smallest gets the value 2, etc. up to the largest difference, which is assigned the value n', if there are n' non-zero differences. If two or more of the differences are the same, they each receive the average of the ranks these values would have received if they had not been tied. Under the null hypothesis of no difference, the sums of the ranks relating to the positive and negative differences should be the same.

---

1 Define the null and alternative hypotheses under study
H_0: the median difference in the population equals zero
H_1: the median difference in the population does not equal zero.

2 Collect relevant data from two related samples

3 Calculate the value of the test statistic specific to H_0
Calculate the difference for each pair of results. Rank all n' non-zero differences, assigning the value 1 to the smallest difference and the value n' to the largest. Sum the ranks of the positive (T_+) and negative differences (T_-).
- If $n' \leq 25$, the test statistic, T, takes the value T_+ or T_-, whichever is smaller.
- If $n' > 25$, calculate the test statistic z, where:

$$z = \frac{\left| T - \dfrac{n'(n'+1)}{4} \right| - \dfrac{1}{2}}{\left(\dfrac{n'(n'+1)(2n'+1)}{24} \right)}$$

which follows a Normal distribution (its value has to be adjusted if there are many tied values[1]).

4 Compare the value of the test statistic to values from a known probability distribution
- If $n' \leq 25$, refer T to Appendix A8
- If $n' > 25$, refer z to Appendix A1

5 Interpret the P-value and results
Interpret the P-value and calculate a confidence interval for the median difference (Topic 19).

Examples

Ninety-six new recruits, all men aged between 16 and 20 years, had their teeth examined when they enlisted in the Royal Air Force. After receiving the necessary treatment to make their teeth dentally fit, they were examined one year later. A complete mouth, excluding wisdom teeth, has 28 teeth and, in this study, every tooth had four sites of periodontal interest; each recruit had a minimum of 84 and a maximum of 112 measurable sites on each occasion. It was of interest to examine the effect of treatment on pocket depth, a measure of gum disease (greater pocket depth indicates worse disease).

As pocket depth (taking the average over the measurable sites in a mouth) was approximately Normally distributed in this sample of recruits, a **paired t-test** was performed to determine whether the average pocket depth was the same before and after treatment. Full computer output is shown in Appendix C.

---

[1] Siegel, S. & Castellan, N.J. (1988) *Nonparametric Statistics for the Behavioural Sciences*, 2nd edn, McGraw-Hill, New York.

1 H_0: the mean difference in a man's average pocket depth before and after treatment in the population of recruits equals zero

H_1: the mean difference in a man's average pocket depth before and after treatment in the population of recruits does not equal zero.

2 Sample size, $n = 96$. Mean difference of average pocket depth, $\bar{d} = 0.1486$ mm. Standard deviation of differences, $s_d = 0.5601$ mm.

3 Test statistic, $t = \dfrac{0.1486}{0.5601/\sqrt{96}} = 2.60$

4 We refer t to Appendix A2 with $(96 - 1) = 95$ degrees

of freedom: $0.01 < P < 0.05$ (computer output gives $P = 0.011$).

5 We have evidence to reject the null hypothesis, and can infer that a recruit's average pocket depth was reduced after treatment. The 95% confidence interval for the true mean difference in average pocket depth is 0.035 to 0.262 mm (i.e. $0.1486 \pm 1.95 \times 0.5601/\sqrt{96}$). Of course, we have to be careful here if we want to conclude that it is the treatment that has reduced average pocket depth, as we have no control group of recruits who did not receive treatment. The improvement may be a consequence of time or a change in dental hygiene habits, and may not be due to the treatment received.

The data in the table below show the percentage of measurable sites for which there was loss of attachment at each assessment in each of 14 of these recruits who were sent to a particular air force base. Loss of attachment is an indication of gum disease that may be more advanced than that assessed by pocket depth. As the differences in the percentages were not Normally distributed, we performed a **Wilcoxon signed ranks test** to investigate whether treatment had any effect on loss of attachment.

1 H_0: the median of the differences (before and after treatment) in the percentages of sites with loss of attachment equals zero in the population of recruits

H_1: the median of the differences in the percentages of sites with loss of attachment does not equal zero in the population.

2 The percentages of measurable sites with loss of attachment, before and after treatment, for each recruit are shown in the table below.

Recruit	1	2	3	4	5	6	7	8	9	10	11	12	13	14
Before (%)	65.5	75.0	87.2	97.1	100.0	92.6	82.3	90.0	93.0	100.0	91.7	97.7	79.0	95.4
After (%)	100.0	10.0	100.0	97.1	99.1	100.0	91.6	94.6	95.5	97.3	92.3	98.0	100.0	99.0
Difference (%)	−34.5	65.0	−12.8	0.0	0.9	−7.4	−9.3	−4.6	−2.5	2.7	−0.6	−0.3	−21.0	−3.6
Rank	12	13	10	—	3	8	9	7	4	5	2	1	11	6

3 There is one zero difference; of the remaining $n' = 13$ differences, three are positive and 10 are negative. The sum of the ranks of the positive differences, $T_+ = 3 + 5 + 13 = 21$.

4 As $n' < 25$, we refer T_+ to Appendix A8: $P > 0.05$.

5 There is insufficient evidence to reject the null hypothesis of no change in the percentage of sites with loss of attachment. The median difference in the percentage of sites with loss of attachment is −3.1% (i.e. the mean of −2.5% and 3.6%), a negative median difference

indicating that, on average, the percentage of sites with loss of attachment is greater *after* treatment, although this difference is not significant. Appendix A7 shows that the approximate 95% confidence interval for the median difference in the population is given by the 3rd and the 12th ranked differences (including the zero difference); these are −21.0% and 0.9%. Although the result of the test is not significant, the lower limit indicates that the percentage of sites with loss of attachment could be as much as 21.0% more after the recruit received treatment!

Duffy, S. (1997) Results of a three year longitudinal study of early periodontitis in a group of British male adolescents. MSc Dissertation, University of London, Eastman Dental Institute for Oral Health Care Sciences.

21 Numerical data: two unrelated groups

The problem
We have samples from two independent (unrelated) groups of individuals and one numerical or ordinal variable of interest. We are interested in whether the mean or distribution of the variable is the same in the two groups. For example, we may wish to compare the weights in two groups of children, each child being randomly allocated to receive either a dietary supplement or placebo.

The unpaired (two-sample) *t*-test
Assumptions
In the population, the variable is Normally distributed and the variances of the two groups are the same. In addition, we have reasonable sample sizes so that we can check the assumptions of Normality and equal variances.

Rationale
We consider the difference in the means of the two groups. Under the null hypothesis that the population means in the two groups are the same, this difference will equal zero. Therefore, we use a test statistic that is based on the difference in the two sample means, and on the value of the difference in population means under the null hypothesis (i.e. zero). This test statistic, often referred to as *t*, follows the *t*-distribution.

Notation
Our two samples are of size n_1 and n_2. Their means are $\bar{x}_1$ and $\bar{x}_2$; their standard deviations are s_1 and s_2.

---

1 Define the null and alternative hypotheses under study

H_0: the population means in the two groups are equal
H_1: the population means in the two groups are not equal.

2 Collect relevant data from two samples of individuals

3 Calculate the value of the test statistic specific to H_0
If s is an estimate of the pooled standard deviation of the two groups,

$$s = \sqrt{\frac{(n_1 - 1)s_1^2 + (n_2 - 1)s_2^2}{n_1 + n_2 - 2}}$$

then the test statistic is given by t where:

continued

$$t = \frac{(\bar{x}_1 - \bar{x}_2) - 0}{SE(\bar{x}_1 - \bar{x}_2)} = \frac{(\bar{x}_1 - \bar{x}_2)}{s\sqrt{\frac{1}{n_1} + \frac{1}{n_2}}}$$

which follows the *t*-distribution with $(n_1 + n_2 - 2)$ degrees of freedom

4 Compare the value of the test statistic to values from a known probability distribution
Refer *t* to Appendix A2. When the sample sizes in the two groups are large, the *t*-distribution approximates a Normal distribution, and then we reject the null hypothesis at the 5% level if the absolute value (i.e. ignoring the sign) of *t* is greater than 1.96.

5 Interpret the *P*-value and results
Interpret the *P*-value and calculate a confidence interval for the difference in the two means. The 95% confidence interval is given by:

$$(\bar{x}_1 - \bar{x}_2) \pm t_{0.05} \times SE(\bar{x}_1 - \bar{x}_2)$$

where $t_{0.05}$ is the percentage point of the *t*-distribution with $(n_1 + n_2 - 2)$ degrees of freedom which gives a two-tailed probability of 0.05.

Interpretation of the confidence interval
The upper and lower limits of the confidence interval can be used to assess whether the difference between the two mean values is clinically important. For example, if the lower limit is close to zero, this indicates that the true difference may be very small and clinically meaningless, even if the test is statistically significant.

If the assumptions are not satisfied
When the sample sizes are reasonably large, the *t*-test is fairly robust (Topic 32) to departures from Normality. However, it is less robust to unequal variances. There is a modification of the unpaired *t*-test that allows for unequal variances, and results from it are often provided in computer output. However, if you are concerned that the assumptions are not satisfied, then you either transform the data (Topic 9) to achieve approximate Normality and/or equal variances, or use a non-parametric test such as the Wilcoxon rank sum test.

The Wilcoxon rank sum (two-sample) test

Rationale

The **Wilcoxon rank sum test** makes no distributional assumptions and is the non-parametric equivalent to the unpaired t-test. The test is based on the sum of the ranks of the values in each of the two groups; these should be comparable after allowing for differences in sample size if the groups have similar distributions. An equivalent test, known as the **Mann–Whitney U test**, gives identical results although it is slightly more complicated to carry out by hand.

---

1 Define the null and alternative hypotheses under study

H_0: the two groups have the same distribution in the population

H_1: the two groups have different distributions in the population.

2 Collect relevant data from two samples of individuals

3 Calculate the value of the test statistic specific to H_0

All observations are ranked as if they were from a single sample. Tied observations are given the average of the ranks the values would have received if they had not been tied. The sum of the ranks, T, is then calculated in the group with the smaller sample size.

- If the sample size in each group is 15 or less, T is the test statistic.
- If at least one of the groups has a sample size of more than 15, calculate the test statistic

$$z = \frac{(T - \mu_T)}{\sigma_T}$$

which follows a Normal distribution, where

$$\mu_T = \frac{n_S(n_S + n_L + 1)}{2} \qquad \sigma_T = \sqrt{n_L \mu_T / 6}$$

and n_S and n_L are the sample sizes of the smaller and larger groups, respectively. z must be adjusted if there are many tied values[1].

4 Compare the value of the test statistic to values from a known probability distribution

- If the sample size in each group is 15 or less, refer T to Appendix A9.
- If at least one of the groups has a sample size of more than 15, refer z to Appendix A1.

5 Interpret the P-value and results

Interpret the P-value and obtain a confidence interval for the difference in the two medians. This is time-consuming to calculate by hand so details have not been included; some statistical packages will provide the CI. If this confidence interval is not included in your package, you can quote a confidence interval for the median in each of the two groups.

Example 1

In order to determine the effect of regular prophylactic inhaled corticosteroids on wheezing episodes associated with viral infection in school age children, a randomized, double-blind controlled trial was carried out comparing inhaled beclomethasone dipropionate with placebo. In this investigation, the primary endpoint was the mean forced expiratory volume (FEV1) over a 6 month period. After checking the assumptions of Normality and constant variance (see Fig. 4.2), we performed an **unpaired t-test** to compare the means in the two groups. Full computer output is shown in Appendix C.

---

1 H_0: the mean FEV1 in the population of school age children is the same in the two treatment groups

H_1: the mean FEV1 in the population of school age children is not the same in the two treatment groups.

2 Treated group: sample size, $n_1 = 50$; mean, $\bar{x}_1 = 1.64$ litres, standard deviation, $s_1 = 0.29$ litres

Placebo group: sample size, $n_2 = 48$; mean, $\bar{x}_2 = 1.54$ litres; standard deviation, $s_2 = 0.25$ litres

3 Pooled standard deviation,

$$s = \sqrt{\frac{(49 \times 0.29^2) + (47 \times 0.25^2)}{(50 + 48 - 2)}} = 0.2670$$

Test statistic, $t = \dfrac{1.64 - 1.54}{0.2670 \times \sqrt{\frac{1}{50} + \frac{1}{48}}} = 1.9145$

continued

---

[1] Siegel, S. & Castellan, N.J. (1988) *Nonparametric Statistics for the Behavioural Sciences*, 2nd edn. McGraw-Hill, New York.

4 We refer t to Appendix A2 with $45 + 48 - 2 = 96$ degrees of freedom. Because Appendix A2 is restricted to certain degrees of freedom, we have to **interpolate** (estimate the required value that lies between two known values). We therefore interpolate between the values relating to 50 and 100 degrees of freedom. Hence, $P > 0.05$ (computer output gives $P = 0.06$).

5 We have insufficient evidence to reject the null hypothesis at the 5% level. However, as the P-value is only just greater than 0.05, there may be an indication that the two population means are different. The estimated difference between the two means is $1.64 - 1.54 = 0.10$ litres. The 95% confidence interval for the true difference in the two means ranges from -0.006 to

$$0.2061 \text{ litres} \left[= 0.10 \pm \left(1.96 \times 0.2670 \times \sqrt{\tfrac{1}{50} + \tfrac{1}{48}} \right) \right].$$

Data kindly provided by Dr I. Doull, Cystic Fibrosis/Respiratory Unit, Department of Child Health, University Hospital of Wales, Cardiff, UK and Ms F.C. Lampe, Department of Primary Care and Population Sciences, Royal Free and University College School of Medicine, Royal Free Campus, London, UK.

Example 2

In order to study whether the mechanisms involved in fatal soybean asthma are different from that of normal fatal asthma, the number of CD3+ T cells in the submucosa, a measure of the body's immune system, was compared in seven cases of fatal soybean dust-induced asthma and 10 fatal asthma cases. Because of the small sample sizes and obviously skewed data, we performed a **Wilcoxon rank sum test** to compare the distributions.

1 H_0: the distributions of CD3+ T-cell numbers in the two groups in the population are the same
H_1: the distributions of CD3+ T-cell numbers in the two groups in the population are not the same.

2 Soy-bean group: sample size, $n = 7$, CD3+ T-cell levels (cells/mm²) were $34.45, 0.00, 1.36, 0.00, 1.43, 0.00, 4.01$
Asthma group: sample size, $n = 10$, CD3+ T-cell levels (cells/mm²) were $74.17, 13.75, 37.50, 1225.51, 99.99, 3.76, 58.33, 73.63, 4.32, 154.86$
The ranked data are shown in the table below.

3 Sum of the ranks in the soy-bean group $= 2 + 2 + 2 + 4 + 5 + 7 + 10 = 32$
Sum of the ranks in the asthma group $= 6 + 8 + 9 + 11 + 12 + 13 + 14 + 15 + 16 + 17 = 121$.

4 Because there are 10 or less values in each group, we obtain the P-value from Appendix A9: $P < 0.01$ (computer output gives $P = 0.003$).

5 There is evidence to reject the null hypothesis that the distributions of CD3+ T-cell levels are the same in the two groups. The median number of CD3+ T cells in the soybean and fatal asthma groups are 1.36 (95% confidence interval 0 to 34.45) and $(58.33 + 73.63)/2 = 65.98$ (95% confidence interval 4.32 to 154.86) cells/mm², respectively. We thus believe that CD3+ T cells are reduced in fatal soybean asthma, suggesting a different mechanism from that described for most asthma deaths.

Soy-bean	0.00	0.00	0.00	1.36	1.43		4.01		34.45							
Asthma						3.76		4.32	13.75	37.50	58.33	73.63	74.17	99.99	154.86	1225.51
Rank	2	2	2	4	5	6	7	8	9	10	11	12	13	14	15	16	17

Data kindly provided by Dr M. Synek, Coldeast Hospital, Sarisbury, and Ms F.C. Lampe, Department of Primary Care and Population Sciences, Royal Free and University College School of Medicine, Royal Free Campus, London UK.

The problem

We have samples from a number of independent groups. We have a single numerical or ordinal variable and are interested in whether the values of the variable vary between the groups, e.g. whether platelet counts vary between women of different ethnic backgrounds. Although we could perform tests to compare the values in each pair of groups, the high Type I error rate, resulting from the large number of comparisons, means that we may draw incorrect conclusions (Topic 18). Therefore, we carry out a single **global** test to determine whether there are differences between any groups.

One-way analysis of variance

Assumptions

The groups are defined by the *levels* of a single factor (e.g. different ethnic backgrounds). In the population of interest, the variable is Normally distributed and the variance in each group is the same. We have a reasonable sample size so that we can check these assumptions.

Rationale

The one-way analysis of variance separates the total variability in the data into that which can be attributed to differences between the individuals from the different groups (the **between-group variation**), and to the random variation between the individuals within each group (the **within-group variation**, sometimes called **unexplained** or **residual** variation). These components of variation are measured using variances, hence the name **analysis of variance** (ANOVA). Under the null hypothesis that the group means are the same, the between-group variance will be similar to the within-group variance. If, however, there are differences between the groups, then the between-group variance will be larger than the within-group variance. The test is based on the ratio of these two variances.

Notation

We have k independent samples, each defining a different group. The sample sizes, means and standard deviations in each group are n_i, $\bar{x}_i$ and s_i, respectively ($i = 1, 2, \ldots, k$). The total sample size is $n = n_1 + n_2 + \ldots + n_k$.

1 Define the null and alternative hypotheses under study

H_0: all group means in the population are equal
H_1: at least one group mean in the population differs from the others.

2 Collect relevant data from samples of individuals

3 Calculate the value of the test statistic specific to H_0

The test statistic for ANOVA is a ratio, F, of the between-group variance to the within-group variance. This F-statistic follows the F-distribution (Topic 8) with $(k - 1)$, $(n - 1)$ degrees of freedom in the numerator and denominator, respectively.

The calculations involved in ANOVA are complex and are not shown here. Most computer packages will output the values directly in an ANOVA table, which usually includes the F-ratio and P-value (see Example).

4 Compare the value of the test statistic to values from a known probability distribution

Refer the F-ratio to Appendix A5. Because the between-group variation is $\geqslant$ the within-group variation, we look at the one-sided P-values.

5 Interpret the P-value and results

If we obtain a significant result at this initial stage, we may consider performing specific pairwise ***post-hoc*** comparisons. We can use one of a number of special tests devised for this purpose (e.g. **Duncan's**, **Scheffé's**) or we can use the unpaired t-test (Topic 21) adjusted for multiple hypothesis testing (Topic 18). We can also calculate a confidence interval for each individual group mean (Topic 11). Note that we use a pooled estimate of the variance of the values from *all* groups when calculating confidence intervals and performing t-tests. Most packages refer to this estimate of the variance as the **residual variance** or **residual mean square**; it is found in the ANOVA table.

Although the two tests appear to be different, the unpaired t-test and ANOVA give equivalent results when there are only two groups of individuals.

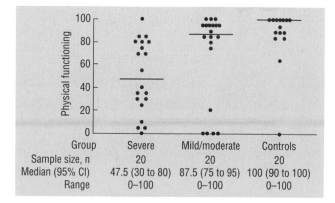

Group	Severe	Mild/moderate	Controls
Sample size, n	20	20	20
Median (95% CI)	47.5 (30 to 80)	87.5 (75 to 95)	100 (90 to 100)
Range	0–100	0–100	0–100

Fig. 22.1 Dot plot showing physical functioning scores (from the SF-36 questionnaire) in individuals with severe and mild/moderate haemophilia and in normal controls. The horizontal bars are the medians.

If the assumptions are not satisfied

Although ANOVA is relatively robust (Topic 32) to moderate departures from Normality, it is not robust to unequal variances. Therefore, before carrying out the analysis, we check for Normality, and test whether the variances are similar in the groups either by eyeballing them, or by using **Levene's** test or **Bartlett's** test (Topic 32). If the assumptions are not satisfied, we can either transform the data (Topic 9), or use the non-parametric equivalent of one-way ANOVA, the Kruskal–Wallis test.

The Kruskal–Wallis test
Rationale

This non-parametric test is an extension of the Wilcoxon rank sum test (Topic 21). Under the null hypothesis of no differences in the distributions between the groups, the sums of the ranks in each of the k groups should be comparable after allowing for any differences in sample size.

[1] Siegel, S. & Castellan, N.J. (1988) *Nonparametric Statistics for the Behavioral Sciences.* McGraw-Hill, New York.

---

1 Define the null and alternative hypotheses under study

H_0: each group has the same distribution of values in the population

H_1: each group does not have the same distribution of values in the population.

2 Collect relevant data from samples of individuals

3 Calculate the value of the test statistic specific to H_0

Rank all n values and calculate the sum of the ranks in each of the groups: these sums are $R_1, \ldots R_k$. The test statistic (which should be modified if there are many tied values[1]) is given by:

$$H = \frac{12}{n(n+1)} \sum \frac{R_i^2}{n_i} - 3(n+1)$$

which follows a Chi-squared distribution with $(k-1)$ df

4 Compare the value of the test statistic to values from a known probability distribution

Refer H to Appendix A3.

5 Interpret the P-value and results

Interpret the P-value and, if significant, perform two-sample non-parametric tests, adjusting for multiple testing. Calculate a confidence interval for the median in each group.

We use one-way ANOVA when the groups relate to a single factor and are independent. We can use other forms of ANOVA when the study design is more complex[2].

[2] Hand, D.J. & Taylor, C.C. (1987) *Multivariate Analysis of Variance and Repeated Measures.* Chapman and Hall, London.

Example 1

A total of 150 women of different ethnic backgrounds were included in a cross-sectional study of factors related to blood clotting. We compared mean platelet levels in the four groups using a **one-way ANOVA**. The assumptions (Normality, constant variance) were met, as shown in the computer output (Appendix C).

1 H_0: there are no differences in the mean platelet levels in the four groups in the population

H_1: at least one group mean platelet level differs from the others in the population

2 The following table summarizes the data in each group.

continued

Group	Sample size n (%)	Mean ($\times 10^9$) $\bar{x}$	Standard deviation ($\times 10^9$), s	95% CI for mean (using pooled standard deviation – see point 3)
Caucasian	90 (60.0)	268.1	77.08	252.7 to 283.5
Afro-Caribbean	21 (14.0)	254.3	67.50	220.9 to 287.7
Mediterranean	19 (12.7)	281.1	71.09	245.7 to 316.5
Other	20 (13.3)	273.3	63.42	238.9 to 307.7

3 The following ANOVA table is extracted from the computer output:

Source	Sums of squares	df	Mean square	F-ratio	P-value
Between ethnic group	7711.967	3	2570.656	0.477	0.6990
Within ethnic group	787289.533	146	5392.394		

Pooled standard deviation $= \sqrt{5392.394} \times 10^9 = 73.43 \times 10^9$.

4 The ANOVA table gives $P = 0.70$. (We could have referred F to Appendix A5 with (3, 146) degrees of freedom to determine the P-value.)

5 There is insufficient evidence to reject the null hypothesis that the mean levels in the four groups in the population are the same.

Data kindly provided by Dr R.A. Kadir, University Department of Obstetrics and Gynaecology, and Professor C.A. Lee, Haemophilia Centre and Haemostasis Unit, Royal Free Hospital, London, UK.

Example 2

Quality-of-life scores, measured using the SF-36 questionnaire, were obtained in three groups of individuals: those with severe haemophilia, those with mild/moderate haemophilia, and normal controls. Each group comprised a sample of 20 individuals. Scores on the physical functioning scale (PFS), which can take values from 0 to 100, were compared in the three groups. As visual inspection of Fig. 22.1 showed that the data were not Normally distributed, we performed a **Kruskal–Wallis** test.

1 H_0: each group has the same distribution of PFS scores in the population

H_1: at least one of the groups has a different distribution of PFS scores in the population.

2 The data are shown in Fig. 22.1.

3 Sum of ranks in severe haemophilia group = 372
Sum of ranks in mild/moderate haemophilia group = 599
Sum of ranks in normal control group = 859

$$H = \frac{12}{60(60+1)}\left(\frac{372^2}{20} + \frac{599^2}{20} + \frac{859^2}{20}\right) - 3(60+1) = 19.47$$

4 We refer H to Appendix A3: $P < 0.001$.

5 There is substantial evidence to reject the null hypothesis that the distribution of PFS scores is the same in the three groups. Pairwise comparisons were carried out using Wilcoxon rank sum tests, adjusting the P-values for the number of tests performed. The individuals with severe and mild/moderate haemophilia both had significantly lower PFS scores than the controls ($P = 0.0003$ and $P = 0.03$, respectively) but the distributions of the scores in the haemophilia groups were not significantly different from each other ($P = 0.09$).

Data kindly provided by Mr A. Miners, Department of Primary Care and Population Sciences, Royal Free and University College Medical School, Royal Free Campus, London, UK, and Dr C. Jenkinson, Health Services Research Unit, University of Oxford, Oxford, UK.

23 Categorical data: a single proportion

The problem

We have a single sample of n individuals; each individual either 'possesses' a characteristic of interest (e.g. is male, is pregnant, has died) or does not possess that characteristic (e.g. is female, is not pregnant, is still alive). A useful summary of the data is provided by the **proportion** of individuals with the characteristic. We are interested in determining whether the true proportion in the population of interest takes a particular value.

The test of a single proportion

Assumptions

Our sample of individuals is selected from the population of interest. Each individual either has or does not have the particular characteristic.

Notation

r individuals in our sample of size n have the characteristic. The estimated proportion with the characteristic is $p = r/n$. The proportion of individuals with the characteristic in the population is π. We are interested in determining whether π takes a particular value, π_1.

Rationale

The number of individuals with the characteristic follows the Binomial distribution (Topic 8), but this can be approximated by the Normal distribution, providing np and $n(1 - p)$ are each greater than 5. Then p is approximately Normally distributed with an estimated mean = p and an estimated standard deviation = $\sqrt{\dfrac{p(1-p)}{n}}$. Therefore, our test statistic, which is based on p, also follows the Normal distribution.

---

1 Define the null and alternative hypotheses under study

H_0: the population proportion, π, is equal to a particular value, π_1

H_1: the population proportion, π, is not equal to π_1.

2 Collect relevant data from a sample of individuals

3 Calculate the value of the test statistic specific to H_0

continued

$$z = \frac{|p - \pi_1| - \dfrac{1}{2n}}{\sqrt{\dfrac{p(1-p)}{n}}}$$

which follows a Normal distribution.

The $1/2n$ in the numerator is a **continuity correction**: it is included to make an allowance for the fact that we are approximating the discrete Binomial distribution by the continuous Normal distribution.

4 Compare the value of the test statistic to values from a known probability distribution

Refer z to Appendix A1.

5 Interpret the P-value and results

Interpret the P-value and calculate a confidence interval for the true population proportion, π. The 95% confidence interval for π is:

$$p \pm 1.96 \sqrt{\frac{p(1-p)}{n}}$$

We can use this confidence interval to assess the clinical or biological importance of the results. A wide confidence interval is an indication that our estimate has poor precision.

The sign test applied to a proportion

Rationale

The sign test (Topic 19) can be used if the response of interest can be expressed as a **preference** (e.g. in a cross-over trial, patients may have a preference for either treatment A or treatment B). If there is no preference overall, then we would expect the proportion preferring A, say, to equal $1/_2$. We use the sign test to assess whether this is so.

Although this formulation of the problem and its test statistic appear to be different from those of Topic 19, both approaches to the sign test produce the same result.

1 Define the null and alternative hypotheses under study

H_0: the proportion, π, of preferences for A in the population is equal to $\frac{1}{2}$

H_1: the proportion of preferences for A in the population is not equal to $\frac{1}{2}$.

2 Collect relevant data from a sample of individuals

3 Calculate the value of the test statistic specific to H_0

Ignore any individuals who have no preference and reduce the sample size from n to n' accordingly. Then $p = r/n'$, where r is the number of preferences for A.

- If $n' \le 10$, count r, the number of preferences for A.
- If $n' > 10$, calculate the test statistic:

$$z' = \frac{\left| p - \frac{1}{2} \right| - \frac{1}{2n'}}{\sqrt{\dfrac{p(1-p)}{n'}}}$$

z' follows the Normal distribution. Note that this formula is based on the test statistic, z, used in the previous box to test the null hypothesis that the population proportion equals π_1; here we replace n by n', and π_1 by $\frac{1}{2}$.

4 Compare the value of the test statistic to values from a known probability distribution

- If $n' \le 10$, refer r to Appendix A6
- If $n' > 10$, refer z' to Appendix A1.

5 Interpret the P-value and results

Interpret the P-value and calculate a confidence interval for the proportion of preferences for A in the entire sample of size n.

Example

Human herpes-virus 8 (HHV-8) has been linked to Kaposi's sarcoma, primary effusion lymphoma and certain types of multicentric Castleman's disease. It has been suggested that HHV-8 can be transmitted sexually. In order to assess the relationships between sexual behaviour and HHV-8 infection, the prevalence of antibodies to HHV-8 was determined in a group of 271 homo/bisexual men attending a London sexually transmitted disease clinic. In the blood donor population in the UK, the seroprevalence of HHV-8 has been documented to be 2.7%. Initially, the seroprevalence from this study was compared to 2.7% using a **single proportion** test.

1 H_0: the seroprevalence of HHV-8 in the population of homo/bisexual men equals 2.7%

H_1: the seroprevalence of HHV-8 in the population of homo/bisexual men does not equal 2.7%.

2 Sample size, $n = 271$; number who are seropositive to HHV8, $r = 50$

Seroprevalence, $p = 50/271 = 0.185$ (i.e. 18.5%)

3 Test statistic is $z = \dfrac{\left| 0.185 - 0.027 \right| - \dfrac{1}{2 \times 271}}{\sqrt{\dfrac{0.185(1 - 0.185)}{271}}} = 6.62$

4 We refer z to Appendix A1: $P < 0.0001$.

5 There is substantial evidence that the seroprevalence of HHV-8 in homo/bisexual men attending sexually transmitted disease clinics in the UK is higher than that in the blood donor population. The 95% confidence interval for the seroprevalence of HHV-8 in the population of homo/bisexual men is 13.9% to 23.1%, calculated as

$$\left\{ 0.185 \pm 1.96 \times \sqrt{\frac{0.185 \times (1 - 0.185)}{271}} \right\} \times 100\%.$$

Data kindly provided by Drs N.A. Smith, D. Barlow, and B.S. Peters, Department of Genitourinary Medicine, Guy's and St Thomas' NHS Trust, London, and Dr J. Best, Department of Virology, Guy's, King's College and St Thomas's School of Medicine, King's College, London, UK.

Example

In a double-blind cross-over study, 36 adults with perennial allergic rhinitis were treated with subcutaneous injections of either inhalant allergens or placebo, each treatment being given daily for a defined period. The patients were asked whether they preferred the active drug or the placebo. The **sign test** was performed to investigate whether the proportions preferring the two preparations were the same.

1 H_0: the proportion preferring the active preparation in the population equals 0.5

H_1: the proportion preferring the active preparation in the population does not equal 0.5.

2 Of the 36 adults, 27 expressed a preference; 21 preferred the active preparation. Of those with a preference, the proportion preferring the active preparation, p = 21/27 = 0.778.

3 Test statistic is $z' = \dfrac{\left|0.778 - 0.5\right| - \dfrac{1}{2 \times 27}}{\sqrt{\dfrac{0.778(1 - 0.778)}{27}}} = 3.24$

4 We refer z' to Appendix A1: $P = 0.001$

5 There is substantial evidence to reject the null hypothesis that the two preparations are preferred equally in the population. The 95% confidence interval for the true proportion is 0.62 to 0.94, calculated as

$$0.778 \pm 1.96 \times \sqrt{\frac{0.778 \times (1 - 0.778)}{27}}.$$

Therefore, at the very least, we believe that almost two-thirds of individuals in the population prefer the active preparation.

Data adapted from: Radcliffe, M.J., Lampe, F.C., Brostoff, J. (1996) Allergen-specific low-dose immunotherapy in perennial allergic rhinitis: a double-blind placebo-controlled crossover study. *Journal of Investigational Allergology and Clinical Immunology*, **6**, 242–247.

Categorical data: two proportions

The problem

- We have two independent groups of individuals (e.g. homosexual men with and without a history of gonorrhoea). We want to know if the proportions of individuals with a characteristic (e.g. infected with human herpesvirus-8, HHV-8) are the same in the two groups.
- We have two related groups, e.g. individuals may be matched, or measured twice in different circumstances (say, before and after treatment). We want to know if the proportions with a characteristic (e.g. raised test result) are the same in the two groups.

Independent groups: the Chi-squared test

Terminology

The data are obtained, initially, as **frequencies**, i.e. the numbers with and without the characteristic in each sample. A table in which the entries are frequencies is called a **contingency table**; when this table has two rows and two columns it is called a **2 × 2 table**. Table 24.1 shows the **observed** frequencies in the four cells corresponding to each row/column combination, the four **marginal totals** (the frequency in a specific row or column, e.g. $a + b$), and the **overall total**, n. We can calculate (see Rationale) the frequency that we would expect in each of the four cells of the table if H_0 were true (the **expected frequencies**).

Assumptions

We have samples of sizes n_1 and n_2 from two independent groups of individuals. We are interested in whether the proportions of individuals who possess the characteristic are the same in the two groups. Each individual is represented only once in the study. The rows (and columns) of the table are **mutually exclusive**, implying that each individual can belong in only one row and only one column. The usual, albeit conservative, approach requires that the expected frequency in each of the four cells is at least five.

Rationale

If the proportions with the characteristic in the two groups are equal, we can estimate the overall proportion of individuals with the characteristic by $p = (a + b)/n$; we **expect** $n_1 \times p$ of them to be in Group 1 and $n_2 \times p$ to be in Group 2. We evaluate expected numbers without the characteristic similarly. Therefore, *each expected frequency is the product of the two relevant marginal totals divided by the overall total*. A large discrepancy between the observed (O) and the corresponding expected (E) frequencies is an indication that the proportions in the two groups differ. The test statistic is based on this discrepancy.

---

1 Define the null and alternative hypotheses under study

H_0: the proportions of individuals with the characteristic are equal in the two groups in the population

H_1: these population proportions are not equal.

2 Collect relevant data from samples of individuals

3 Calculate the value of the test statistic specific to H_0

$$\chi^2 = \sum \frac{\left(|O - E| - \frac{1}{2}\right)^2}{E}$$

where O and E are the observed and expected frequencies, respectively, in each of the four cells of the table. The vertical lines around $O-E$ indicate that we ignore its sign. The $1/2$ in the numerator is the continuity correction (Topic 19). The test statistic follows the Chi-squared distribution with 1 degree of freedom.

4 Compare the value of the test statistic to values from a known probability distribution

Refer χ^2 to Appendix A3.

5 Interpret the P-value and results

Interpret the P-value and calculate the confidence interval for the difference in the true population proportions. The 95% confidence interval is given by:

$$(p_1 - p_2) \pm 1.96 \sqrt{\frac{p_1(1 - p_1)}{n_1} + \frac{p_2(1 - p_2)}{n_2}}$$

If the assumptions are not satisfied

If $E < 5$ in any one cell, we use **Fisher's exact test** to obtain a P-value that does not rely on the approximation to the Chi-squared distribution. This is best left to a computer program as the calculations are tedious to perform by hand.

Table 24.1 Observed frequencies.

Characteristic	Group 1	Group 2	Total
Present	a	b	$a + b$
Absent	c	d	$c + d$
Total	$n_1 = a + c$	$n_2 = b + d$	$n = a + b + c + d$
Proportion with characteristic	$p_1 = \dfrac{a}{n_1}$	$p_2 = \dfrac{b}{n_2}$	$p = \dfrac{a + b}{n}$

Related groups: McNemar's test

Assumptions

The two groups are related or dependent, e.g. each individual may be measured in two different circumstances. Every individual is classified according to whether the characteristic is present in both circumstances, one circumstance only, or in neither (Table 24.2).

Table 24.2 Observed frequencies of pairs in which the characteristic is present or absent.

	Circumstance 1		
	Present	Absent	Total no. of pairs
Circumstance 2			
Present	w	x	$w + x$
Absent	y	z	$y + z$
Total	$w + y$	$x + z$	$m = w + x + y + z$

Rationale

The observed proportions with the characteristic in the two circumstances are $(w + y)/m$ and $(w + x)/m$. They will differ if x and y differ. Therefore, to compare the proportions with the characteristic, we ignore those individuals who agree in the two circumstances, and concentrate on the discordant pairs, x and y.

---

1 Define the null and alternative hypotheses under study

H_0: the proportions with the characteristic are equal in the two groups in the population

H_1: these population proportions are not equal.

2 Collect relevant data from two samples

3 Calculate the value of the test statistic specific to H_0

$$\chi^2 = \frac{(|x - y| - 1)^2}{x + y}$$

which follows the Chi-squared distribution with 1 degree of freedom. The 1 in the numerator is a continuity correction (Topic 19).

4 Compare the value of the test statistic with values from a known probability distribution
Refer χ^2 to Appendix A3.

5 Interpret the P-value and results
Interpret the P-value and calculate the confidence interval for the difference in the true population proportions. The approximate 95% CI is:

$$\frac{x - y}{m} \pm \frac{1.96}{m}\sqrt{x + y - \frac{(x - y)^2}{m}}$$

Example 1

In order to assess the relationship between sexual risk factors and HHV-8 infection (study described in Topic 23), the prevalence of seropositivity to HHV-8 was compared in homo/bisexual men who had a previous history of gonorrhoea, and those who had not previously had gonorrhoea, using the **Chi-squared test**. A typical computer output is shown in Appendix C.

1 H_0: the seroprevalence rate is the same in those with and without a history of gonorrhoea in the population
   H_1: the seroprevalence rates are not the same in the two groups in the population.

2 The observed frequencies are shown in the following contingency table: 14/43 (32.6%) and 36/228 (15.8%) of those with and without a previous history of gonorrhoea are seropositive for HHV-8, respectively.

3 The expected frequencies are shown in the four cells of the contingency table.
The test statistic is χ^2,

$$\chi^2 = \left\{ \frac{(|14 - 7.93| - \frac{1}{2})^2}{7.93} + \frac{(|36 - 42.07| - \frac{1}{2})^2}{42.07} \right.$$

$$\left. + \frac{(|29 - 35.07| - \frac{1}{2})^2}{35.07} + \frac{(|192 - 185.93| - \frac{1}{2})^2}{185.93} \right\}$$

$$= 5.70$$

4 We refer χ^2 to Appendix A3 with 1 df: $0.01 < P < 0.05$. (Computer output gives $P = 0.017$.)

5 There is evidence of a real difference in the seroprevalence rates in the two groups in the population. We estimate this difference as $32.6\% - 15.8\% = 16.8\%$. The 95% CI for the true difference in the two percentages is 2.0% to 31.6% [i.e. $16.8 \pm 1.96 \times \sqrt{(\{32.6 \times 67.4\}/43 + \{15.8 \times 84.2\}/228)}$].

Continued

HHV-8	Previous history of gonorrhoea				
	Yes		No		
	Observed	Expected	Observed	Expected	Total
Seropositive	14	$(43 \times 50/271)$ $= 7.93$	36	$(228 \times 50/271)$ $= 42.07$	50
Seronegative	29	$(43 \times 221/271)$ $= 35.07$	192	$(228 \times 221/271)$ $= 185.93$	221
Total	43		228		271

Example 2

In order to compare two methods of establishing the cavity status (present or absent) of teeth, a dentist assessed the condition of 100 first permanent molar teeth that had either tiny or no cavities using radiographic techniques. These results were compared with those obtained using the more objective approach of visually assessing a section of each tooth. The percentages of teeth detected as having cavities by the two methods of assessment were compared using **McNemar's test**.

1 H_0: the two methods of assessment identify the same percentage of teeth with cavities in the population
H_1: these percentages are not equal.

2 The frequencies for the matched pairs are displayed in the table:

Diagnosis on section	Radiographic diagnosis		
	Cavities absent	Cavities present	Total
Cavities absent	45	4	49
Cavities present	17	34	51
Total	62	38	100

3 Test statistic, $\chi^2 = \dfrac{(|17 - 4| - 1)^2}{17 + 4} = 6.86$

4 We refer χ^2 to Appendix A3 with 1 degree of freedom: $0.001 < P < 0.01$.

5 There is substantial evidence to reject the null hypothesis that the same percentage of teeth are detected as having cavities using the two methods of assessment. The radiographic method has a tendency to fail to detect cavities. We estimate the difference in percentages of teeth detected as having cavities as $51\% - 38\% = 13\%$. An approximate confidence interval for the true difference in the percentages is given by 4.4% to 21.6%

$$\left(\text{i.e. } \left\{ \frac{|17 - 4|}{100} \pm \frac{1.96}{100} \times \sqrt{(17 + 4) - \frac{(17 - 4)^2}{100}} \right\} \times 100\% \right).$$

Adapted from Ketley, C.E. & Holt, R.D. (1993) Visual and radiographic diagnosis of occlusal caries in first permanent molars and in second primary molars. *British Dental Journal*, **174**,364–370.

25 Categorical data: more than two categories

Chi-squared test: large contingency tables

The problem
Individuals can be classified by two factors. For example, one factor may represent disease severity (mild, moderate or severe) and the other factor may represent blood group (A, B, O, AB). We are interested in whether the two factors are associated. Are individuals of a particular blood group likely to be more severely ill?

Assumptions
The data may be presented in an $r \times c$ contingency table with r rows and c columns (Table 25.1). The entries in the table are **frequencies**; each cell contains the number of individuals in a particular row and a particular column. Every individual is represented once, and can only belong in one row and in one column, i.e. the categories of each factor are mutually exclusive. At least 80% of the expected frequencies are greater than or equal to 5.

Rationale
The null hypothesis is that there is no association between the two factors. Note that if there are only two rows and two columns, then this test of no association is the same as that of two proportions (Topic 24). We calculate the frequency that we expect in each cell of the contingency table if the null hypothesis is true. As explained in Topic 24, the expected frequency in a particular cell is the product of the relevant row total and relevant column total, divided by the overall total. We calculate a test statistic that focuses on the discrepancy between the observed and expected frequencies in every cell of the table. If the overall discrepancy is large, then it is unlikely the null hypothesis is true.

1 Define the null and alternative hypotheses under study

H_0: there is no association between the categories of one factor and the categories of the other factor in the population

H_1: the two factors are associated in the population.

2 Collect relevant data from a sample of individuals

3 Calculate the value of the test statistic specific to H_0

$$\chi^2 = \sum \frac{(O - E)^2}{E}$$

where O and E are the observed and expected frequencies in each cell of the table. The test statistic follows the Chi-squared distribution with degrees of freedom equal to $(r-1) \times (c-1)$.

Because the approximation to the Chi-squared distribution is reasonable if the degrees of freedom are greater than one, we do not need to include a continuity correction (as we did in Topic 24).

4 Compare the value of the test statistic to values from a known probability distribution
Refer χ^2 to Appendix A3.

5 Interpret the P-value and results

If the assumptions are not satisfied
If more than 20% of the expected frequencies are less than 5, we try to combine, appropriately (i.e. so that it makes scientific sense), two or more rows and/or two or more columns of the contingency table. We then recalculate the expected frequencies of this reduced table, and carry on reducing the table, if necessary, to ensure that the $E \geq 5$ condition is satisfied. If we have reduced our table to a 2×2 table so that it can be reduced no further and we still have small expected frequencies, we use Fisher's exact test (Topic 24) to evaluate the exact P-value. Some computer packages will compute Fisher's exact P-values for larger contingency tables.

Chi-squared test for trend

The problem
Sometimes we investigate relationships in categorical data when one of the two factors has only two categories (e.g. the

Table 25.1 Observed frequencies in an $r \times c$ table.

Row categories	Col 1	Col 2	Col 3	...	Col c	Total
Row 1	f_{11}	f_{12}	f_{13}	...	f_{1c}	R_1
Row 2	f_{21}	f_{22}	f_{23}	...	f_{2c}	R_2
Row 3	f_{31}	f_{32}	f_{33}	...	f_{3c}	R_3
...	...	...	...	...	...	...
...	...	...	...	...	...	...
Row r	f_{r1}	f_{r2}	f_{r3}	...	f_{rc}	R_r
Total	C_1	C_2	C_3	...	C_c	n

presence or absence of a characteristic) and the second factor can be categorised into k, say, mutually exclusive categories that are ordered in some sense. For example, one factor might be whether or not an individual responds to treatment, and the ordered categories of the other factor may represent four different age (in years) categories 65–69, 70–74, 75–79 and ≥80. We can then assess whether there is a trend in the proportions with the characteristic over the categories of the second factor. For example, we may wish to know if the proportions responding to treatment tend to increase (say) with increasing age.

Table 25.2 Observed frequencies and assigned scores in a $2 \times k$ table.

Characteristic	Col 1	Col 2	Col 3	...	Col k	Total
Present	f_{11}	f_{12}	f_{13}	...	f_{1k}	R_1
Absent	f_{21}	f_{22}	f_{23}	...	f_{2k}	R_2
Total	C_1	C_2	C_3	...	C_k	n
Score	w_1	w_2	w_3	...	w_k	

---

1 Define the null and alternative hypotheses under study

H_0: there is no trend in the proportions with the characteristic in the population

H_1: there is a trend in the proportions in the population.

continued

---

2 Collect relevant data from a sample of individuals

We estimate the proportions with the characteristic in each of the k categories. We assign a score to each of the column categories. Typically these are the successive values, $1, 2, 3, \ldots, k$, but, depending on how we have classified the column factor, they could be numbers that in some way suggest the relative values of the ordered categories (e.g. the midpoint of the age range defining each category) or the trend we wish to investigate (e.g. linear or quadratic). The use of any equally spaced numbers (e.g. $1, 2, 3, \ldots, k$) allows us to investigate a linear trend.

3 Calculate the value of the test statistic specific to H_0

$$\chi^2 = \frac{\left(\sum w_i f_{1i} - R_1 \sum \frac{w_i C_i}{n} \right)^2}{\frac{R_1}{n}\left(1 - \frac{R_1}{n}\right)\left(\sum C_i w_i^2 - n\left(\sum \frac{w_i C_i}{n} \right)^2 \right)}$$

using the notation of Table 25.2, and where the sums extend over all the k categories. The test statistic follows the Chi-squared distribution with (1) degrees of freedom.

4 Compare the value of the test statistic to values from a known probability distribution

Refer χ^2 to Appendix A3.

5 Interpret the P-value and results

Interpret the P-value and calculate a confidence interval for each of the k proportions (Topic 11).

Example

A cross-sectional survey was carried out among the elderly population living in Southampton, with the objective of measuring the frequency of cardiovascular disease. A total of 259 individuals, ranging between 65 and 95 years of age, were interviewed. Individuals were grouped into four age groups (65–69, 70–74, 75–79 and 80+ years) at the time of interview. We used the **Chi-squared test** to determine whether the prevalence of chest pain differed in the four age groups.

---

1 H_0: there is no association between age and chest pain in the population

H_1: there is an association between age and chest pain in the population.

2 The observed frequencies (%) and expected frequencies are shown in the following table.

continued

3 Test statistic, $\chi^2 = \left[\dfrac{(15-9.7)^2}{9.7} + \ldots + \dfrac{(41-39.1)^2}{39.1} \right]$

$= 4.839$

4 We refer χ^2 to Appendix A3 with 3 degrees of freedom: $P > 0.10$ (computer output gives $P = 0.18$).

5 There is insufficient evidence to reject the null hypothesis of no association between chest pain and age in the population of elderly people. The estimated proportions (95% confidence intervals) with chest pain for the four successive age groups, starting with the youngest, are: 0.20 (0.11, 0.29), 0.12 (0.04, 0.19), 0.10 (0.02, 0.17) and 0.09 (0.02, 0.21).

Chest pain	Age (years)				Total
	65–69	70–74	75–79	80+	
Yes					
Observed	15 (20.3%)	9 (11.5%)	6 (9.7%)	4 (8.9%)	34
Expected	9.7	10.2	8.1	5.9	
No					
Observed	59 (79.7%)	69 (88.5%)	56 (90.3%)	41 (91.1%)	225
Expected	64.3	67.8	53.9	39.1	
Total	74	78	62	45	259

As the four age groups in this study are ordered, it is also possible to analyse these data using a **Chi-squared test for trend**, which takes into account the ordering of the groups. We may obtain a significant result from this test, even though the general test of association gave a non-significant result. We assign the scores of 1, 2, 3 and 4 to each of the four age groups, respectively, and because of their even spacing, can test for a linear trend.

1 H_0: there is no linear association between age and chest pain in the population

H_1: there is a linear association between age and chest pain in the population.

2 The data are displayed in the table above. We assign scores of 1, 2, 3 and 4 to the four age groups, respectively.

3 Test statistic is χ^2.

4 We refer χ^2 to Appendix A3 with 1 degree of freedom: $P > 0.05$ (computer output gives $P = 0.051$).

5 There is only borderline evidence to reject the null hypothesis of no linear association between chest pain and age in the population of elderly people.

$$\chi^2 = \frac{\left\{ [(1 \times 15) + \ldots + (4 \times 4)] - 34 \times \left[\left(\dfrac{1 \times 74}{259} \right) + \ldots + \left(\dfrac{4 \times 45}{259} \right) \right] \right\}^2}{\dfrac{34}{259} \times \left(1 - \dfrac{34}{259}\right) \times \left\{ [(74 \times 1^2) + \ldots + (45 \times 4^2)] - 259 \times \left[\left(\dfrac{1 \times 74}{259} \right) + \ldots + \left(\dfrac{4 \times 45}{259} \right) \right]^2 \right\}} = 3.79$$

Adapted from: Dewhurst, G., Wood, D.A., Walker, F., *et al.* (1991) A population survey of cardiovascular disease in elderly people: design, methods and prevalence results. *Age and Ageing* **20**, 353–360.

26 Correlation

Introduction

Correlation analysis is concerned with measuring the degree of association between two variables, x and y. Initially, we assume that both x and y are **numerical**, e.g. height and weight.

Suppose we have a pair of values, (x, y), measured on each of the n individuals in our sample. We can mark the point corresponding to each individual's pair of values on a two-dimensional **scatter diagram** (Topic 4). Conventionally, we put the x variable on the horizontal axis, and the y variable on the vertical axis in this diagram. Plotting the points for all n individuals, we obtain a scatter of points that may suggest a relationship between the two variables.

Pearson correlation coefficient

We say that we have a **linear relationship** between x and y if a straight line drawn through the midst of the points provides the most appropriate approximation to the observed relationship. We measure how close the observations are to the straight line that best describes their linear relationship by calculating the **Pearson product moment correlation coefficient**, usually simply called the **correlation coefficient**. Its true value in the *population*, ρ (the Greek letter, rho), is estimated in the *sample* by r, where

$$r = \frac{\sum(x - \bar{x})(y - \bar{y})}{\sqrt{\sum(x - \bar{x})^2 \sum(y - \bar{y})^2}}$$

which is usually obtained from computer output.

Properties

- r lies between -1 and $+1$.
- Its **sign** indicates whether one variable increases as the other variable increases (positive r) or whether one variables decreases as the other increases (negative r) (see Fig. 26.1).
- Its **magnitude** indicates how close the points are to the straight line. In particular if $r = +1$ or -1, then there is perfect correlation with all the points lying on the line (this is most unusual, in practice); if $r = 0$, then there is no **linear** correlation (although there may be a non-linear relationship). The closer r is to the extremes, the greater the degree of linear association (Fig. 26.1).
- It is dimensionless, i.e. it has no units of measurement.
- Its value is valid only within the range of values of x and y in the sample. You cannot infer that it will have the same value when considering values of x or y that are more extreme than the sample values.
- x and y can be interchanged without affecting the value of r.

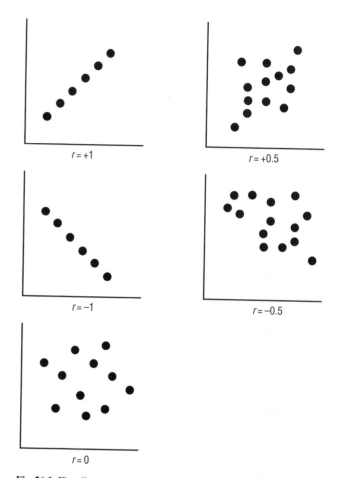

Fig. 26.1 Five diagrams indicating values of r in different situations.

- A correlation between x and y does not necessarily imply a 'cause and effect' relationship.
- r^2 represents the proportion of the variability of y that can be attributed to its linear relationship with x (Topic 28).

When not to calculate r

It may be misleading to calculate r when:
- there is a non-linear relationship between the two variables (Fig. 26.2a), e.g. a quadratic relationship (Topic 30);
- when the data include more than one observation on each individual;
- in the presence of outliers (Fig. 26.2b);
- the data comprise subgroups of individuals for which the mean levels of the observations on at least one of the variables are different (Fig. 26.2c).

Hypothesis test for the Pearson correlation coefficient

We want to know if there is any linear correlation between two numerical variables. Our sample consists of n independent pairs of values of x and y. We assume that at least one of the two variables is Normally distributed.

---

1 Define the null and alternative hypotheses under study

$H_0: \rho = 0$
$H_1: \rho \neq 0$

2 Collect relevant data from a sample of individuals

3 Calculate the value of the test statistic specific to H_0

Calculate r.

- If $n \leq 200$, r is the test statistic

- If $n > 200$, calculate $T = \sqrt{\dfrac{(n-2)}{(1-r^2)}}$

which follows a t-distribution with $n - 2$ degrees of freedom.

4 Compare the value of the test statistic to values from a known probability distribution

If $n \leq 150$, refer r to Appendix A10.
If $n > 150$, refer T to Appendix A2.

5 Interpret the P-value and results

Calculate a confidence interval for ρ. Provided *both variables are approximately Normally distributed*, the approximate 95% confidence interval for ρ is:

$$\left(\frac{e^{2z_1} - 1}{e^{2z_1} + 1}, \frac{e^{2z_2} - 1}{e^{2z_2} + 1} \right)$$

where $z_1 = z - \dfrac{1.96}{\sqrt{n-3}}$, $z_2 = z + \dfrac{1.96}{\sqrt{n-3}}$, and

$z = 0.5 \log_e \left[\dfrac{(1+r)}{(1-r)} \right]$.

Note that, if the sample size is large, H_0 may be rejected even if r is quite close to zero. Alternatively, even if r is large, H_0 may not be rejected if the sample size is small. For this reason, it is particularly helpful to calculate r^2, the proportion of the total variance explained by the relationship. For example, if $r = 0.40$ then $P < 0.05$ for a sample size of 25, but the relationship is only explaining 16% (= $0.40^2 \times 100$) of the variability of one variable.

Spearman's rank correlation coefficient

We calculate **Spearman's rank correlation coefficient**, the non-parametric equivalent to Pearson's correlation coefficient, if one or more of the following points is true:

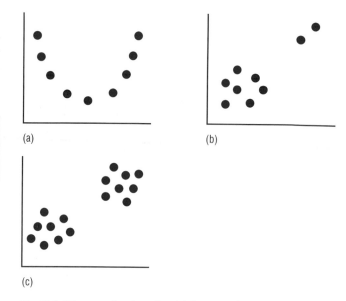

(a)   (b)

(c)

Fig. 26.2 Diagrams showing when it is inappropriate to calculate the correlation coefficient. (a) Relationship not linear, $r = 0$. (b) In the presence of outlier(s). (c) Data comprise subgroups.

- at least one of the variables, x or y, is measured on an ordinal scale;
- neither x nor y is Normally distributed;
- the sample size is small;
- we require a measure of the association between two variables when their relationship is non-linear.

Calculation

To estimate the population value of Spearman's rank correlation coefficient, ρ_s, by its sample value, r_s:

1 Arrange the values of x in increasing order, starting with the smallest value, and assign successive *ranks* (the numbers 1, 2, 3, ..., n) to them. Tied values receive the average of the ranks these values would have received had there been no ties.

2 Assign ranks to the values of y in a similar manner.

3 r_s is the Pearson's correlation coefficient between the *ranks* of x and y.

Properties and hypothesis tests

These are the same as for Pearson's correlation coefficient, replacing r by r_s, except that:

- r_s provides a measure of association (not necessarily linear) between x and y;
- when testing the null hypothesis that $\rho_s = 0$, refer to Appendix A11 if the sample size is less than or equal to 10;
- we do not calculate r_s^2 (it does not represent the proportion of the total variation in one variable that can be attributed to its relationship with the other).

Example

As part of a study to investigate the factors associated with changes in blood pressure in children, information was collected on demographic and lifestyle factors, and clinical and anthropometric measures in 4245 children aged from 5 to 7 years. The relationship between height (cm) and systolic blood pressure (mmHg) in a sample of 100 of these children is shown in the scatter diagram (Fig. 28.1); there is a tendency for taller children in the sample to have higher blood pressures. **Pearson's correlation coefficient** between these two variables was investigated. Appendix C contains a computer output from the analysis.

---

1 H_0: the population value of the Pearson correlation coefficient, ρ, is zero

H_1: the population value of the Pearson correlation coefficient is not zero.

2 We can show (Fig. 34.1) that the sample values of both height and systolic blood pressure are approximately Normally distributed.

3 We calculate r as 0.33. This is the test statistic since $n \leq 200$.

4 We refer r to Appendix A10 with a sample size of 100: $P < 0.001$.

5 There is strong evidence to reject the null hypothesis; we conclude that there is a linear relationship between systolic blood pressure and height in the population of such children. However, $r^2 = 0.33 \times 0.33 = 0.11$. Therefore, despite the highly significant result, the relationship between height and systolic blood pressure explains only a small percentage, 11%, of the variation in systolic blood pressure.

In order to determine the 95% confidence interval for the true correlation coefficient, we calculate:

$$z = 0.5\ln\left(\frac{1.33}{0.67}\right) = 0.3428$$

$$z_1 = 0.3428 - \frac{1.96}{9.849} = 0.1438$$

$$z_2 = 0.3428 + \frac{1.96}{9.849} = 0.5418$$

Thus the confidence interval ranges from

$$\frac{(e^{2 \times 0.1438} - 1)}{(e^{2 \times 0.1438} + 1)} \text{ to } \frac{(e^{2 \times 0.5418} - 1)}{(e^{2 \times 0.5418} + 1)}, \text{i.e. from } \frac{0.33}{2.33} \text{ to } \frac{1.96}{3.96}.$$

We are thus 95% certain that ρ lies between 0.14 and 0.49.

As we might expect, given that each variable is Normally distributed, **Spearman's rank correlation coefficient** between these variables gave a comparable estimate of 0.32. To test $H_0: \rho_s = 0$, we refer this value to Appendix A10 and again find $P < 0.001$.

Data kindly provided by Ms O. Papacosta and Dr P. Whincup, Department of Primary Care and Population Sciences, Royal Free and University College Medical School, Royal Free Campus, London, UK.

27 The theory of linear regression

What is linear regression?

To investigate the relationship between two continuous variables, x and y, we measure the values of x and y on each of the n individuals in our sample. We plot the points on a **scatter diagram** (Topics 4 and 26), and say that we have a **linear** relationship if the data approximate a straight line. If we believe y is dependent on x, with a change in y being attributed to a change in x, rather than the other way round, we can determine the **linear regression line** (the **regression of y on x**) that best describes the straight line relationship between the two variables.

The regression line

The mathematical equation which estimates the **simple linear regression** line is:

$$Y = a + bx$$

- x is called the **independent**, **predictor** or **explanatory** variable;
- for a given value of x, Y is the value of y (called the **dependent**, **outcome** or **response** variable), which lies on the estimated line. It is the value we *expect* for y (i.e. its average) if we know the value of x, and is called the **fitted** value of y;
- a is the **intercept** of the estimated line; it is the value of Y when $x = 0$ (Fig. 27.1);
- b is the **slope** or **gradient** of the estimated line; it represents the amount by which Y increases on average if we increase x by one unit (Fig. 27.1).

a and b are called the **regression coefficients** of the estimated line, although this term is often reserved only for b. We show how to evaluate these coefficients in Topic 28. Simple linear regression can be extended to include more than one explanatory variable; in this case, it is known as **multiple linear regression** (Topic 29).

Method of least squares

We perform regression analysis using a sample of observations. a and b are the sample estimates of the true parameters, α and β, which define the linear regression line in the population. a and b are determined by the **method of least squares** in such a way that the 'fit' of the line $Y = a + bx$ to the points in the scatter diagram is optimal. We assess this by considering the **residuals** (the vertical distance of each point from the line, i.e. **residual = observed y – fitted Y**, Fig. 27.2). The **line of best fit** is chosen so that the sum of the *squared* residuals is a *minimum*.

Assumptions

1 There is a linear relationship between x and y

2 The observations in the sample are independent. The observations are independent if there is no more than one pair of observations on each individual.

3 For each value of x, there is a distribution of values of y in the population; this distribution is Normal. The mean of this distribution of y values lies on the true regression line (Fig. 27.3).

4 The variability of the distribution of the y values in the population is the same for all values of x, i.e. the variance, σ^2, is constant (Fig. 27.3).

5 The x variable can be measured without error. Note that we do not make any assumptions about the distribution of the x variable.

Many of the assumptions which underlie regression analysis relate to the distribution of the y population for a specified value of x, but they may be framed in terms of the residuals. It is easier to check the assumptions (Topic 28) by studying the residuals than the values of y.

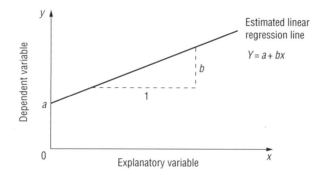

Fig. 27.1 Linear regression line showing the intercept, a, and the slope, b (the increase in Y for a unit increase in x).

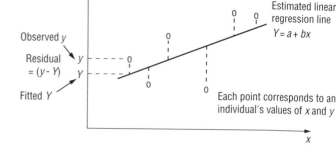

Fig. 27.2 Linear regression line showing the residual (vertical dotted line) for each point.

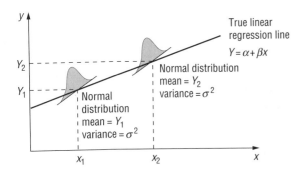

Fig. 27.3 Illustration of assumptions made in linear regression.

Analysis of variance table

Description
Usually the computer output in a regression analysis contains an **analysis of variance table**. In analysis of variance (Topic 22), the total variation of the variable of interest, in this case 'y', is partitioned into its component parts. Because of the linear relationship of y on x, we expect y to vary as x varies; we call this the variation which is **due to** or **explained by the regression**. The remaining variability is called the **residual error** or **unexplained** variation. The residual variation should be as small as possible; if so, most of the variation in y will be explained by the regression, and the points will lie close to the line; i.e. the line is a **good fit**.

Purposes
The analysis of variance table enables us to do the following.

1 Assess how well the line fits the data points. From the information provided in the table, we can calculate the proportion of the total variation in y that is explained by the regression. This proportion, usually expressed as a percentage and denoted by R^2 (in simple linear regression it is r^2, the square of the correlation coefficient; Topic 26), allows us to assess subjectively the **goodness-of-fit** of the regression equation.

2 Test the **null hypothesis** that the true slope of the line, β, is zero; a significant result indicates that there is evidence of a linear relationship between x and y.

3 Obtain an estimate of the **residual variance**. We need this for testing hypotheses about the slope or the intercept, and for calculating confidence intervals for these parameters and for predicted values of y.

We provide details of the more common procedures in Topic 28.

Regression to the mean
The statistical use of the word 'regression' derives from a phenomenon known as **regression to the mean**, attributed to Sir Francis Galton in 1889. He demonstrated that although tall fathers tend to have tall sons, the average height of the sons is less than that of their tall fathers. The average height of the sons has 'regressed' or 'gone back' towards the mean height of all the fathers in the population. So, on average, tall fathers have shorter (but still tall) sons and short fathers have taller (but still short) sons.

We observe regression to the mean in **screening** and in **clinical trials**, when a subgroup of patients may be selected for treatment because their levels of a certain variable, say cholesterol, are extremely high (or low). If the measurement is repeated some time later, the average value for the second reading for the subgroup is usually less than that of the first reading, tending towards (i.e. regressing to) the average of the age- and sex-matched population, irrespective of any treatment they may have received. Patients recruited into a clinical trial on the basis of a high cholesterol level on their first examination are thus likely to show a drop in cholesterol levels on average at their second examination, even if they remain untreated during this period.

28 Performing a linear regression analysis

The linear regression line

After selecting a sample of size n from our population, and drawing a **scatter diagram** to confirm that the data approximate a straight line, we estimate the **regression of y on x** as:

$$Y = a + bx$$

where Y is the fitted or predicted value of y, a is the intercept, and b is the slope that represents the average change in Y for a unit change in x (Topic 27).

Drawing the line

To draw the line $Y = a + bx$ on the scatter diagram, we choose three values of x, x_1, x_2 and x_3, along its range. We substitute x_1 in the equation to obtain the corresponding value of Y, namely $Y_1 = a + bx_1$; Y_1 is our **fitted** value for x_1 which corresponds to the **observed** value, y_1. We repeat the procedure for x_2 and x_3 to obtain the corresponding values of Y_2 and Y_3. We plot these points on the scatter diagram and join them to produce a straight line.

Checking the assumptions

For each observed value of x, the **residual** is the observed y minus the corresponding fitted Y. Each residual may be either positive or negative. We can use the residuals to check the following assumptions underlying linear regression.

1 There is a linear relationship between x and y: *Either* plot y against x (the data should approximate a straight line), *or* plot the residuals against x (we should observe a random scatter of points rather than any systematic pattern).

2 The observations are independent: the observations are independent if there is no more than one pair of observations on each individual.

3 The residuals are Normally distributed with a mean of zero: Draw a histogram, stem-and-leaf plot, box-and-whisker plot (Topic 4) or Normal plot (Topic 32) of the residuals and 'eyeball' the result.

4 The residuals have the same variability (constant variance) for all the fitted values of y: Plot the residuals against the fitted values, Y, of y; we should observe a random scatter of points. If the scatter of residuals progressively increases or decreases as Y increases, then this assumption is not satisfied.

5 The x variable can be measured without error.

Failure to satisfy the assumptions

If the linearity, Normality and/or constant variance assumptions are in doubt, we may be able to transform x or y (Topic 9), and calculate a new regression line for which these assumptions are satisfied. It is not always possible to find a satisfactory transformation. The linearity and independence assumptions are the most important. If you are dubious about the Normality and/or constant variance assumptions, you may proceed, but the P-values in your hypothesis tests, and the estimates of the standard errors, may be affected. Note that the x variable is rarely measured without any error; provided the error is small, this is usually acceptable because the effect on the conclusions is minimal.

Outliers and influential points

- An **outlier** is a value that is inconsistent with most of the values in the data set (Topic 3). We can often detect outliers by looking at the scatter diagram or the residual plots.
- An **influential point** has the effect of substantially altering the estimates of the slope and the intercept of the regression line when it is included in the analysis. If formal methods of detection are not available, you may have to rely on intuition; you should recalculate the regression line without the point and note the effect.

Do not discard outliers or influential points routinely because their omission may affect your conclusions. Always investigate the reasons for their presence and report them.

Assessing goodness-of-fit

We can judge how well the line fits the data by calculating R^2 (usually expressed as a percentage), which is equal to the square of the correlation coefficient (Topics 26 and 27). This represents the proportion or percentage of the variability of y that can be **explained** by its relationship with x. Its compliment, $(100 - R^2)$, represents the percentage of the variation in y that is **unexplained** by the relationship. There is no formal test to assess R^2; we have to rely on subjective judgement to evaluate the fit of the regression line.

Investigating the slope

If the slope of the line is zero, there is no linear relationship between x and y: changing x has no effect on y. There are two approaches, with identical results, to **testing the null hypothesis that the true slope, β, is zero**.

- *Examine the F-ratio* (equal to the ratio of the 'explained' to the 'unexplained' mean squares) in the analysis of variance table. It follows the F-distribution and has $(1, n - 2)$ degrees of freedom in the numerator and denominator, respectively.

- *Calculate the test statistic* $= \dfrac{b}{SE(b)}$ which follows the t-distribution on $n - 2$ degrees of freedom, where $\text{SE}(b)$ is the standard error of b.

In either case, a significant result, usually if $P < 0.05$, leads to rejection of the null hypothesis.

We calculate the **95% confidence interval** for β as $b \pm t_{0.05}\,\mathrm{SE}(b)$, where $t_{0.05}$ is the percentage point of the t-distribution with $n - 2$ degrees of freedom which gives a two-tailed probability of 0.05. It is the interval that contains the true slope with 95% certainty. For large samples, say $n > 45$, we can approximate $t_{0.05}$ by 1.96.

Regression analysis is rarely performed by hand; computer output from most statistical packages will provide all of this information.

Using the line for prediction

We can use the regression line for predicting values of y for values of x within the observed range (never extrapolate beyond these limits). We predict the mean value of y for individuals who have a certain value of x by substituting that value of x into the equation of the line. So, if $x = x_0$, we predict y as $Y_0 = a + bx_0$. We use this predicted value, and its standard error, to evaluate the confidence interval for the true mean value of y in the population. Repeating this procedure for various values of x allows us to construct confidence limits for the line. This is a band or region that contains the true line with, say, 95% certainty. Similarly, we can calculate a wider region within which we expect most (usually 95%) of the *observations* to lie.

Useful formulae for hand calculations

$$\bar{x} = \sum x / n \quad \text{and} \quad \bar{y} = \sum y / n$$

$$a = \bar{y} - b\bar{x}$$

$$b = \frac{\sum (x - \bar{x})(y - \bar{y})}{\sum (x - \bar{x})^2}$$

$$s_{\mathrm{res}}^2 = \frac{\sum (y - Y)^2}{(n - 2)}, \text{ the estimated residual variance}$$

$$\mathrm{SE}(b) = \frac{s_{\mathrm{res}}}{\sqrt{\sum (x - \bar{x})^2}}$$

Example

The relationship between height (measured in cm) and systolic blood pressure (SBP, measured in mmHg) in the children described in Topic 26 is shown in Fig. 28.1. We performed a **simple linear regression analysis** of systolic blood pressure on height. Assumptions underlying this analysis are verified in Figs 28.2 to 28.4. A typical computer output is shown in Appendix C. There is a significant linear relationship between height and systolic blood pressure, as can be seen by the significant F-ratio in the analysis of variance table in Appendix C ($F = 12.03$ with 1 and 98 degrees of freedom in the numerator and denominator, respectively, $P = 0.0008$). The R^2 of the model is 10.9%. Only approximately a tenth of the variability in the

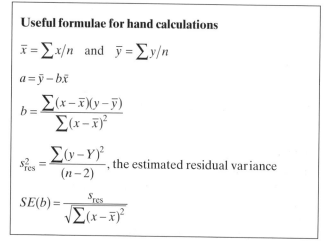

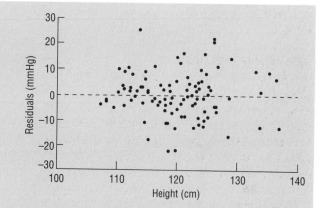

Fig. 28.2 No relationship is apparent in this diagram, indicating that a linear relationship between height and systolic blood pressure is appropriate.

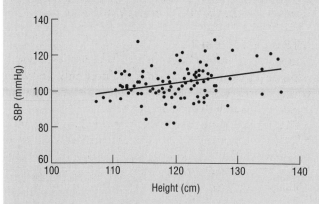

Fig. 28.1 Scatter plot showing relationship between systolic blood pressure (SBP) and height. The estimated regression line, SBP = $46.28 + 0.48 \times$ height, is marked on the scatter plot.

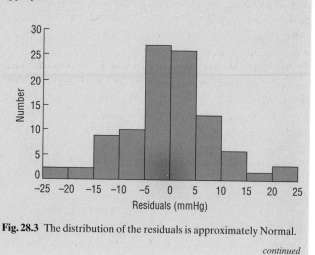

Fig. 28.3 The distribution of the residuals is approximately Normal.

continued

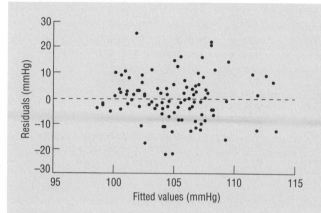

Fig. 28.4 There is no tendency for the residuals to increase or decrease systematically with the fitted values. Hence the constant variance assumption is satisfied.

systolic blood pressure can thus be explained by the model; that is, by differences in the heights of the children. The computer output provides the following information:

Variable	Parameter estimate	Standard Error	Test statistic	*P*-value
Intercept	46.2817	16.7845	2.7574	0.0070
Height	0.4842	0.1396	3.4684	0.0008

The parameter estimate for 'Intercept' corresponds to *a*, and that for 'Height' corresponds to *b* (the slope of the regression line). So, the equation of the estimated regression line is:

$$SBP = 46.28 + 0.48 \times \text{height}$$

In this example, the intercept is of no interest in its own right (it relates to the predicted blood pressure for a child who has a height of zero centimetres—clearly out of the range of values seen in the study). However, we can interpret the slope coefficient; in these children, systolic blood pressure is predicted to increase by 0.48 mmHg, on average, for each centimetre increase in height.

$P = 0.0008$ for the hypothesis test for height (i.e. H_0: true slope equals zero) is identical to that obtained from the analysis of variance table in Appendix C, as expected.

A 95% confidence interval can be calculated for the true slope. This is given by:

$$b \pm 1.96 \times SE(b) = 0.48 \pm (1.96 \times 0.14)$$

Therefore, the 95% confidence interval for the slope ranges from 0.21 to 0.75 mmHg per cm increase in height. This confidence interval does not include zero, confirming the finding that the slope is significantly different from zero.

We can use the regression equation to predict the systolic blood pressure we expect a child of a given height to have. For example, a child who is 115 cm tall has a predicted systolic blood pressure of 46.28 + (0.48 × 115) = 101.48 mmHg; a child who is 130 cm tall has a predicted systolic blood pressure of 46.28 + (0.48 × 130) = 108.68 mm Hg.

What is it?

We may be interested in the effect of several explanatory variables, $x_1, x_2, \ldots, x_k$, on a response variable, y. If we believe that these x's may be inter-related, we should not look, in isolation, at the effect on y of changing the value of a single x, but should simultaneously take into account the values of the other x's. For example, as there is a strong relationship between a child's height and weight, we may want to know whether the relationship between height and systolic blood pressure (Topic 28) is changed when we take the child's weight into account. Multiple linear regression allows us to investigate the joint effect of these explanatory variables on y. Note that, although the explanatory variables are sometimes called independent variables, this is a misnomer because they may be related.

We take a sample of n individuals, and measure the value of each of the variables on every individual. The multiple linear regression equation which estimates the relationships in the population is:

$$Y = a + b_1 x_1 + b_2 x_2 + \ldots + b_k x_k$$

- x_i is the ith explanatory variable or **covariate** ($i = 1, 2, 3, \ldots, k$);
- Y is the predicted, expected or fitted value of y, which corresponds to a particular set of values of $x_1, x_2, \ldots, x_k$;
- a is the constant term, sometimes called the intercept; it is the value of y when all the x's are zero;
- $b_1, b_2, \ldots, b_k$ are the estimated **partial regression coefficients**; b_1 represents the amount by which y increases on average if we increase x_1 by one unit but keep all the other x's constant (i.e. **adjust** for them). If there is a relationship between x_1 and the other x's, b_1 differs from the estimate of the regression coefficient obtained by regressing y on only x_1, because the latter approach does not adjust for the other variables. b_1 represents the effect of x_1 on y that is **independent** of the other xs.

Invariably, you will perform a multiple regression analysis on the computer, and so we omit the formulae for these estimated parameters.

Why do it?

To be able to:
- determine the extent to which each of the explanatory variables is linearly related to the dependent variable, after adjusting for the other variables;
- predict the value of the dependent variable from the explanatory variables.

Assumptions

The assumptions in multiple regression are the same (if we replace 'x' by 'each of the x's') as those in simple linear regression (Topic 27), and are checked in the same way. Failure to satisfy the linearity or independence assumptions is particularly important. We can transform (Topic 9) the y variable and/or some or all of the x variables if the assumptions are in doubt, and then repeat the analysis (including checking the assumptions) on the transformed data.

Categorical explanatory variables

We can perform a multiple regression analysis using *categorical* explanatory variables. In particular, if we have a **binary** variable, x_1 (e.g. male = 0, female = 1), and we increase x_1 by one unit, we are 'changing' from males to females. b_1 thus represents the difference in the estimated mean values of y between females and males, after adjusting for the other x's.

If we have a **nominal** explanatory variable that has more than two categories of response (Topic 1), we have to create a number of new (**dummy**) binary variables[1]. Some computer packages will do this automatically. However, if we have an **ordinal** explanatory variable and its three or more categories can be assigned values on a meaningful linear scale (e.g. social classes 1–5), then we can use these values directly in the multiple regression equation.

Analysis of covariance

An extension of analysis of variance (ANOVA, Topic 22) is the **analysis of covariance**, in which we compare the response of interest between groups of individuals (e.g. two or more treatment groups) when other variables measured on each individual are taken into account. Such data can be analysed using multiple regression techniques by creating one or more binary variables to differentiate between the groups. So, if we wish to compare the average values of y in two treatment groups, while controlling for the effect of variables, $x_2, x_3, \ldots, x_k$ (e.g. age, weight, ...), we create a binary variable, x_1, to represent 'treatment' (e.g. $x_1 = 0$ for treatment A, $x_1 = 1$ for treatment B). In the multiple regression equation, b_1 is the estimated difference in the mean responses on y between treatments B and A, adjusting for the other x's.

Choice of explanatory variables

As a rule of thumb, we should not perform a multiple regression analysis if the number of variables is greater

[1] Armitage, P. & Berry, G. (1994) *Statistical Methods in Medical Research*, 3rd edn. Blackwell Scientific Publications, Oxford.

than the number of individuals divided by 10. Most computer packages have automatic procedures for selecting variables, e.g. stepwise selection (Topic 31). These are particularly useful when many of the explanatory variables are related. A particular problem arises when **collinearity** is present, i.e. when pairs of explanatory variables are extremely highly correlated, and the standard errors of their partial regression coefficients are very large. Then we may find that a group of very highly correlated variables explains much of the variability in the response variable (as judged by R^2), even though each partial regression coefficient in the group is non-significant. In this situation, caution is suggested when interpreting the results.

Analysis

Most computer output contains the following items.

1 An assessment of goodness-of-fit

The **adjusted R^2** represents the proportion of the variability of y which can be explained by its relationship with the x's. R^2 is adjusted so that models with different numbers of explanatory variables can be compared. If it has a low value (judged subjectively), the model is a poor fit. Goodness-of-fit is particularly important when we use the multiple regression equation for prediction.

2 The F-test in the ANOVA table

This tests the null hypothesis that all the partial regression coefficients in the population, $\beta_1, \beta_2, \dots, \beta_k$, are zero. A significant result indicates that there is a linear relationship between y and at least one of the x's.

3 The t-test of each partial regression coefficient, β_i ($i = 1, 2, \dots, k$)

Each t-test relates to one explanatory variable, and is relevant if we want to determine whether that explanatory variable affects the response variable, while controlling for the effects of the other covariates. To test H_0: $\beta_i = 0$, we calculate the test statistic $= \dfrac{b_i}{SE(b_i)}$, which follows the t-distribution with (n – *number of explanatory variables* – *1*) degrees of freedom. Computer output includes the values of each b_i, $SE(b_i)$ and the related test statistic with its P-value. Sometimes the 95% confidence interval for β_i is included; if not, it can be calculated as $b_i \pm t_{0.05} SE(b_i)$.

Example

In Topic 28, we studied the relationship between systolic blood pressure and height in 100 children. It is known that height and weight are positively correlated. We therefore performed a **multiple regression analysis** to investigate the effects of height (cm), weight (kg) and sex (0 = boy, 1 = girl) on systolic blood pressure (mmHg) in these children. Assumptions underlying this analysis are verified in Figs 29.1 to 29.4.

A typical output from a computer analysis of these data is contained in Appendix C. The analysis of variance table indicates that at least one of the explanatory variables is related to systolic blood pressure ($F = 14.95$ with 3 and 96 degrees of freedom in the numerator and denominator, respectively, $P = 0.0001$). The adjusted R^2 value of 0.2972 indicates that 29.7% of the variability in systolic blood pressure can be explained by the model—that is, by differences in the height, weight *and* sex of the children. Thus this provides a much better fit to the data than the simple

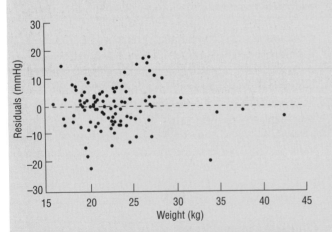

Fig. 29.1 There is no systematic pattern to the residuals when plotted against weight. (Note that, similarly to Fig. 28.2, a plot of the residuals from this model against height also shows no systematic pattern).

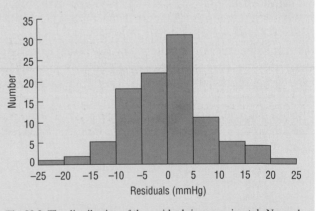

Fig. 29.2 The distribution of the residuals is approximately Normal and the variance is slightly less than that from the simple regression model (Topic 28), reflecting the improved fit of the multiple regression model over the simple model.

continued

linear regression in Topic 28 in which $R^2 = 0.11$. Typical computer output contains the following information about the explanatory variables in the model:

Variable	Parameter estimate	Standard error	95% CI for parameter	Test statistic	P-value
Intercept	79.4395	17.1182	(45.89 to 112.99)	4.6406	0.0001
Height	−0.0310	0.1717	(−0.37 to 0.31)	−0.1807	0.8570
Weight	1.1795	0.2614	(0.67 to 1.69)	4.5123	0.0001
Sex	4.2295	1.6105	(1.07 to 7.39)	2.6261	0.0101

The multiple regression equation is given by:

$$SBP = 79.44 - (0.03 \times height) + (1.18 \times weight) + (4.23 \times sex)$$

The relationship between weight and systolic blood pressure is highly significant ($P < 0.0001$), with a one kilogram increase in weight being associated with an average increase of 1.18 mmHg in systolic blood pressure, after adjusting for height and sex. However, after adjusting for the weight and sex of the child, the relationship between height and systolic blood pressure becomes non-significant ($P = 0.86$). This suggests that the significant relationship between height and systolic blood pressure in the simple regression analysis reflects the fact that taller children tend to be heavier than shorter children. There is a significant relationship ($P = 0.01$) between sex and systolic blood pressure; systolic blood pressure in girls tends to be 4.23 mmHg higher, on average, than that of boys, even after taking account of possible differences in height and weight. Hence, both weight and sex are independent predictors of a child's systolic blood pressure.

We can calculate the systolic blood pressures we would expect for children of given heights and weights. If the first child mentioned in Topic 28 who is 115 cm tall is a girl and weighs 37 kg, she now has a predicted systolic blood pressure of $79.44 - (0.03 \times 115) + (1.18 \times 37) + (4.23 \times 1) = 123.88$ mmHg (higher than the 101.48 mmHg predicted in Topic 28); if the second child who is 130 cm tall is a boy and weighs 30 kg, he now has a predicted systolic blood pressure of $79.44 - (0.03 \times 130) + (1.18 \times 30) + (4.23 \times 0) = 110.94$ mmHg (higher than the 108.68 mmHg predicted in Topic 28).

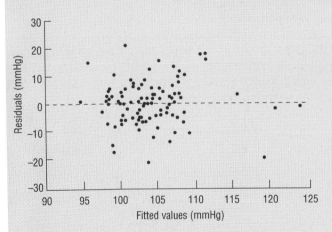

Fig. 29.3 As with the univariate model, there is no tendency for the residuals to increase or decrease systematically with fitted values. Hence the constant variance assumption is satisfied.

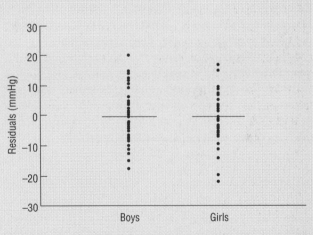

Fig. 29.4 The distribution of the residuals is similar in boys and girls, suggesting that the model fits equally well in the two groups.

30 Polynomial and logistic regression

Polynomial regression

When we plot y against x, we may find that a linear relationship is not appropriate, and that a polynomial (e.g. quadratic, cubic) relationship is preferable. We can modify a multiple regression equation (Topic 29) to accommodate polynomial regression. We just introduce terms into the equation that represent the relevant higher orders of x. So, for example, if we have a cubic relationship, our estimated equation is $Y = a + b_1x + b_2x^2 + b_3x^3$. Usually, the polynomial regression equation will include the highest power of x deemed appropriate (e.g. x^3 for a cubic relationship) and all lower powers of x (i.e. x and x^2 for a cubic relationship). We fit this model, and proceed with the analysis in exactly the same way as if the quadratic and cubic terms represented different variables (x_2 and x_3, say) in a multiple regression analysis. For example, we may fit a cubic model that comprises the explanatory 'variables' height, height^2 and height^3.

Logistic regression
Reasoning

Logistic regression is very similar to linear regression; we use it when we have a **binary dependent variable** (e.g. the presence/absence of a symptom, or an individual who does/does not have a disease) and a number of explanatory variables. We want to know which explanatory variables influence the outcome, and can then use the equation to predict the outcome category into which an individual will fall from values of his/her explanatory variables.

We start by creating a binary variable to represent the two outcomes of the dependent variable (e.g. $y = 1$ designates 'has disease', $y = 0$ designates 'does not have disease'). As this variable is binary, the assumptions underlying linear regression are not met. Furthermore, we cannot interpret predicted values that are not equal to zero or one. So, instead, we predict the probability, p, that an individual will be classified into a particular category of outcome, say 'has disease'. To overcome mathematical difficulties, we use the **logistic** or **logit** transformation (Topic 9) of p in the logistic equation. The logit of this probability is the natural logarithm (i.e. to base e) of the **odds of 'disease'**, i.e.

$$\text{logit}(p) = \ln\frac{p}{1-p}.$$

The equation and its interpretation

An iterative process, rather than ordinary least squares regression (so we cannot use linear regression software), produces, from the sample data, an estimated logistic regression equation of the form:

$$\text{Logit}(P) = a + b_1x_1 + b_2x_2 + \dots + b_kx_k$$

- x_i is the ith explanatory variable ($i = 1, 2, 3, \dots, k$);
- $\text{logit}(P)$ is the predicted value of $\text{logit}(p)$;
- a is the constant term;
- $b_1, b_2, \dots, b_k$ are the estimated **logistic regression coefficients**.

We interpret the exponential of a particular coefficient, for example, e^{b1}, as an **odds ratio** (Topic 16). It is the odds of disease when x_1 takes a particular value relative to the odds of disease when x_1 is increased by one unit, while adjusting for all other x's in the equation. The odds ratio is an estimate of **relative risk**. If the relative risk is equal to one (unity), then the 'risks' of having the disease are the same when x_1 increases by one unit. A value of the relative risk above one indicates an increased risk of having the disease, and a value below one indicates a decreased risk of having the disease, as x_1 increases by one unit.

Computer output
For each explanatory variable

Comprehensive computer output for a logistic regression analysis includes, for each explanatory variable, the estimated logistic regression coefficient with standard error, the estimated odds ratio (i.e. the exponential of the coefficient) with a confidence interval for its true value, and a Wald test statistic (testing the null hypothesis that the relative risk of 'disease' associated with this variable is unity) and associated P-value. We use this information to determine whether each variable is related to the outcome of interest (e.g. disease), and to quantify the extent to which this is so. Automatic selection procedures (Topic 31) can be used, as in multiple linear regression, to select the best combination of explanatory variables.

To assess the adequacy of the model

Usually, interest is centred on examining the explanatory variables and their effect on the outcome. This information is routinely available in all advanced statistical computer packages. However, there are inconsistencies between the packages in the way in which the adequacy of the model is assessed, and in the way it is described. Your computer output may contain the following (in one guise or another).
- A quantity called **−2 log likelihood**: it has an approximately Chi-squared distribution, and indicates how poorly the model fits with all the explanatory variables in the model (a significant result indicates poor prediction).

- The **model Chi-square** or the **Chi-square for covariates**: this tests the null hypothesis that all the regression coefficients in the model are zero. A significant result suggests that at least one covariate is significantly associated with the dependent variable. It can be modified to compare models with differing numbers of covariates.
- The percentages of individuals correctly predicted as 'diseased' or 'disease-free' by the model. This information may be in a **classification table**.

- A **histogram**: this has the predicted probabilities along the horizontal axis, and uses symbols (such as 1 and 0) to designate the group ('diseased' or 'disease-free') to which an individual belongs. A good model will separate the symbols into two groups which show little or no overlap.
- **Indices of predictive efficiency**: these are not routinely available in every computer package. Our advice is to refer to more advanced texts for further information[1].

Example

In a study of the relationship between human herpesvirus type 8 (HHV-8) infection (described in Topic 23) and sexual behaviour, 271 homo/bisexual men were asked questions relating to their past history of a number of sexually transmitted diseases (gonorrhoea, syphilis, herpes simplex type 2 [HSV-2] and HIV). In Topic 24 we showed that men who had a history of gonorrhoea had a higher seroprevalence of HHV-8 than those without a previous history of gonorrhoea. A **multiple logistic regression** analysis was performed to investigate whether this effect was simply a reflection of the relationships between HHV-8 and the other infections and/or the men's age. The explanatory variables were the presence of each of the four infections, each coded as '0' if the patient had no history of the particular infection or '1' if he had a history of that infection, and the patient's age in years.

A typical computer output is displayed in Appendix C. It shows that the Chi-square for covariates equals 24.598 on 5 degrees of freedom ($P = 0.0002$), indicating that at least one of the covariates is significantly associated with HHV-8 serostatus. The table below summarises the information about each variable in the model.

These results indicate that HSV-2 positivity ($P = 0.04$) and HIV status ($P = 0.007$) are independently associated with HHV-8 infection; individuals who are HSV-2 seropositive have 2.21 times (= exp[0.7910]) the risk of

being HHV-8 seropositive as those who are HSV-2 seronegative after adjusting for the other infections. In other words, the risk of HHV-8 seropositivity in these individuals is increased by 121%. The upper limit of the confidence interval for this odds ratio shows that this increased risk could be as much as 371%. HSV-2 infection is a well-documented marker of sexual activity. Thus, rather than HSV-2 being a cause of HHV-8 infection, the association may be a reflection of the sexual activity of the individual.

In addition, there is a tendency for a history of syphilis to be associated with HHV-8 serostatus. Although this is marginally non-significant ($P = 0.09$), we should note that the confidence interval does include values for the odds ratio as high as 13.28. In contrast, there is no indication of an independent relationship between a history of gonorrhoea and HHV-8 seropositivity, suggesting that this variable appeared, by the Chi-squared test (Topic 24), to be associated with HHV-8 serostatus because of the fact that many men who had a history of one of the other sexually transmitted diseases in the past also had a history of gonorrhoea. There is no significant relationship between HHV-8 seropositivity and age; the odds ratio indicates that the risk of HHV-8 seropositivity increases by 0.6% for each additional year of age.

Variable	Parameter estimate	Standard error	Wald Chi-square	P-value	Odds ratio	95% CI for odds ratio
Intercept	−2.2242	0.6512	11.6670	0.0006	—	—
Gonorrhoea	0.5093	0.4363	1.3626	0.2431	1.664	(0.71–3.91)
Syphilis	1.1924	0.7111	2.8122	0.0935	3.295	(0.82–13.28)
HSV-2 positivity	0.7910	0.3871	4.1753	0.0410	2.206	(1.03–4.71)
HIV	1.6357	0.6028	7.3625	0.0067	5.133	(1.57–16.73)
Age	0.0062	0.0204	0.0911	0.7628	1.006	(0.97–1.05)

[1] Menard, S. (1995) Applied logistic regression analysis. In: *Sage University Paper Series on Quantitative Applications in the Social Sciences*, Series no. 07-106. Sage University Press, Thousand Oaks, California.

31 Statistical modelling

Statistical modelling includes the use of simple and multiple linear regression, polynomial regression, logistic regression and methods that deal with survival data. All these methods rely on generating the **mathematical model** that describes the relationship between two or more variables.

In general, any model can be expressed in the form:

$$g(Y) = a + b_1 x_1 + b_2 x_2 + \ldots + b_k x_k$$

where Y is the fitted value of the dependent variable, $g(.)$ is some optional transformation of it (for example, the logit transformation), $x_1, \ldots, x_k$ are the predictor or explanatory variables (which may include polynomial terms or be categorical), $b_1, \ldots, b_k$ are estimated coefficients that relate to these explanatory variables, and a is a constant term.

Model selection

In order for a model to be acceptable, it should be sensible from a clinical standpoint. The inclusion of large numbers of variables in a model, especially those that are highly correlated, may lead to spurious results that are inconsistent with expectations. Therefore, explanatory variables should only be considered for inclusion in the model if there is reason to suppose, from a biological or clinical standpoint, that they are related to the dependent variable.

There is always the danger of **over-fitting** models by including a very large number of explanatory variables. At its extreme, a model is **saturated** when there are as many (or more) variables as individuals. Although explaining the data very well, an over-fitted or saturated model is generally of little use for predicting future outcomes. A usual rule-of-thumb is to ensure that there are at least 10 times as many individuals as explanatory variables.

Often, we have a large number of explanatory variables that we believe may be related to the dependent variable. For example, many factors may appear to be related to systolic blood pressure, including age, dietary and other lifestyle factors. A first step is to assess the relationship between each variable, one-by-one, and the dependent variable, e.g. using simple regression. We then consider, for further investigation, only those explanatory variables that appear to be related to the dependent variable. **Automatic selection procedures**, performed on the computer, provide a means of creating the optimal model, by selecting some of these variables.

- **All subsets**—every combination of explanatory variables is considered; that which provides the best fit, as described by the model R^2 (Topic 27) or some other measure, is selected.
- **Forwards selection**—variables that contribute most to the R^2 of the model are progressively added until no further variable contributes significantly to R^2.
- **Backwards selection**—all possible variables are included. Those that contribute least to R^2 are progressively removed until none of the remaining variables can be removed without leading to significant loss of R^2.
- **Stepwise selection**—a combination of forwards and backwards selection that starts by progressing forwards and then, at the end of each 'step', checks backwards to ensure that all of the included variables are still required.

Although these procedures remove much of the manual aspect of model selection, they have some disadvantages. First, it is possible that two or more models will fit the data equally well, leading to different conclusions. Second, the resulting models, although mathematically justifiable, may not be sensible. Therefore, a combination of these procedures and common sense should be applied when selecting the best fitting model.

Numerical explanatory variables

When a **numerical explanatory variable**, x, is added to a model it is usually assumed that the relationship between the dependent variable, y, and that variable is linear, i.e. there is a straight line relationship between the two variables. However, a polynomial relationship (Topic 30), or some other non-linear relationship, may be more appropriate.

- **Numerical dependent variable**: we show in Topic 32 how to check for linearity. If the relationship is not linear, then either we take a transformation of one or other or the variables (e.g. by taking logs, Topic 9) or categorize the explanatory variable (Topic 29) before including it in the model.
- **Binary dependent variable** ($y = 0$ or 1): we can check for linearity by categorizing individuals into groups according to their values of the explanatory variable; we observe whether a linear trend is present in the proportions with a specific outcome ($y = 1$, say) in each group (Topic 25).

Prognostic indices and risk scores for a binary response

Given a large number of demographic or clinical features of an individual, we may want to *predict* whether that individual is likely to develop disease. Models, often fitted using proportional hazards regression (Topic 41), logistic regression (Topic 30) or a similar method known as **discriminant analysis**, can be used to identify factors that are significantly associated with outcome. A **prognostic index** or **risk score** can then be generated from the coefficients of this model, and the score calculated for an individual to assess his/her likelihood of disease. However, a model that explains a large proportion of the variability in the data may not necessarily be good at predicting which patients will develop disease. Therefore, once we have derived a predictive score based on a model, we should assess the **validity** of that score.

Validating the score

We can validate our score in a number of ways.
• We produce a prediction table based on our data set, showing the number of individuals in whom we correctly and incorrectly predict the disease status (similar to the table in Topic 35). Measures, including sensitivity and specificity, can be calculated for this table, *or*
• We categorize individuals according to their score and consider disease rates in the different categories (see Example); we should see a relationship between the categories and disease rates, e.g. with higher scored categories having greater disease rates.

Clearly, any model will always perform well on the data set that was used to generate the model. Therefore, in order to provide a true assessment of the usefulness of the score, it should be validated on other, independent, data sets.

Where this is impractical, we may separate the data into two roughly equally sized sub-samples. The first sub-sample, known as the **training sample**, is used to generate the model. The second sub-sample, known as the **validation sample**, is used for validating the results from the training sample. As a consequence of the smaller sample size, fewer explanatory variables can be included in the model.

Jackknifing

This is a way of both estimating and validating a score in an unbiased manner. Each individual is removed from the sample, one at a time, and the remaining $(n - 1)$ individuals are used to estimate the parameters of the model. This process is repeated for each of the n individuals in the sample, and the results are averaged over all n samples. Because this score is generated from many different data sets, it can be validated on the complete data set without taking sub-samples.

Example

Although there are wide differences in prognosis between patients with AIDS, they are often thought of as a single homogeneous group. In order to group patients correctly according to their likely prognosis, a prognostic score was generated on the basis of the clinical experience of 363 AIDS patients at a single centre in London. A total of 159 (43.8%) of these patients died over a follow-up period of 6 years.

The score was the weighted sum of the number of each type (mild, moderate or severe) of AIDS-defining diseases the patient had experienced and his/her minimum CD4 cell count (measured in cells/mm^3) and was equal to:

Score = 300 × number of very severe AIDS events (lymphoma)
+100 × number of severe AIDS events (all events, other than those listed as very severe or mild)
+20 × number of mild AIDS events (oesophageal candida, cutaneous Kaposi's sarcoma, *Pneumocystis carinii* pneumonia, extrapulmonary tuberculosis)
−1 × minimum CD4 cell count measured since AIDS

In order to aid the interpretation of this score, and to validate it, three groups were identified.

AIDS Grade I   Score < 0
AIDS Grade II   Score 0–99
AIDS Grade III Score ≥ 100

Validation of the score was assessed by considering the death rate (number of deaths divided by the total person-years of follow-up) in each grade.

AIDS grade	Deaths	Follow-up (person-years)	Death rate
I	17	168.0	1.0
II	54	153.9	3.5
III	71	81.2	8.7

Thus there is a clear trend towards increasing death rates as the score increases. The score was also validated on a group of patients from a second London centre.

AIDS grade	Deaths	Follow-up (person-years)	Death rate
I	65	828.5	0.8
II	229	579.6	4.0
III	322	361.3	8.9

Remarkably similar results were seen, thus confirming the value of this scoring system.

Adapted from: Mocroft, A.J., Johnson, M.A., Sabin, C.A., *et al.* (1995) Staging system for clinical AIDS patients. Lancet **346**; 12–17.

32 Checking assumptions

Why bother?

Computer analysis of data offers the opportunity of handling large data sets that might otherwise be beyond our capabilities. However, do not be tempted to 'have a go' at statistical analyses simply because they are available on the computer. The validity of the conclusions drawn rely on the appropriate analysis being conducted in any given circumstance, and a requirement that the underlying assumptions inherent in the proposed statistical analysis are satisfied. We say that an analysis is **robust** to violations of its assumptions if its *P*-value and power (Topic 18) are not appreciably affected by the violations. Performing a non-robust analysis could lead to misleading conclusions.

Are the data Normally distributed?

Many analyses make assumptions about the underlying distribution of the data. The following procedures verify approximate Normality, the most common of the distributional assumptions.

• We produce a dot plot (for small samples) or a histogram, stem-and-leaf plot (Fig. 4.2) or box plot to show the empirical frequency distribution of the data (Topic 4). We conclude that the distribution is approximately Normal if it is bell-shaped and symmetrical. The median in a box plot should cut the rectangle defining the first and third quartiles in half, and the two whiskers should be of equal length if the data are Normally distributed.

• Alternatively, we can produce a **Normal plot** (preferably on the computer) which plots the cumulative frequency distribution of the data (on the horizontal axis) against that of the Normal distribution. Lack of Normality is indicated by the resulting plot producing a curve that appears to deviate from a straight line (Fig. 32.1).

Although both approaches are subjective, the Normal plot is more effective for smaller samples. The **Kolmogorov-Smirnov** and **Shapiro-Wilk** tests, both performed on the computer, can be used to assess Normality more objectively.

Are two or more variances equal?

We explained how to use the *t*-test (Topic 21) to compare two means, and ANOVA (Topic 22) to compare more than two means. Underlying these analyses is the assumption that the variability of the observations in each group is the same, i.e. we require equal variances, described as **homogeneity of variance** or **homoscedasticity**. We have **heterogeneity of variance** if the variances are unequal.

• We can use **Levene's test**, using a computer program, to test for homogeneity of variance in two or more groups. The null hypothesis is that all the variances are equal. Levene's

test has the advantage that it is not strongly dependent on the assumption of Normality. **Bartlett's test** can also be used to compare more than two variances, but it is non-robust to departures from Normality.

• We can use the *F*-**test (variance-ratio test)** described in the box to compare two variances, provided the data in each group are approximately Normally distributed (the test is non-robust to a violation of this assumption). The two estimated variances are s_1^2 and s_2^2, calculated from n_1 and n_2 observations, respectively. By convention, we choose s_1^2 to be the larger of the two variances, if they differ.

---

1 Define the null and alternative hypotheses under study

H_0: the two population variances are equal
H_1: the two population variances are unequal.

2 Collect relevant data from a sample of individuals

3 Calculate the value of the test statistic specific to H_0

$$F = s_1^2/s_2^2$$

which follows an *F*-distribution with $n_1 - 1$ *df* in the numerator, and $n_2 - 1$ *df* in the denominator. By choosing $s_1^2 \geq s_2^2$, we have ensured that the *F*-ratio will always be ≥ 1. This allows us to use the tables of the *F*-distribution, which are tabulated only for values ≥ 1.

4 Compare the value of the test statistic to values from a known probability distribution

Refer *F* to Appendix A5. Our two-sided alternative hypothesis leads to a two-tailed test.

5 Interpret the *P*-value and results

Note that we are rarely interested in the variances *per se*, so we do not usually calculate confidence intervals for them.

Are variables linearly related?

Most of the techniques which we discussed in Topics 26–30 assume that there is a linear (straight line) relationship between two or, sometimes, more than two variables. Any inferences drawn from such analyses rely on the linearity assumption being satisfied. The simplest way of checking for linearity between two variables is to plot one variable against the other, and 'eyeball' the resulting scatter of points which should broadly follow a straight line. Alternatively, we can plot the residuals against the values of the explanatory variable (x); we should observe a random scatter of points (Fig. 28.2).

What if the assumptions are not satisfied?

We have various options.
- Proceed as planned, recognizing that this may result in a non-robust analysis. Be aware of the implications if you do this. Do not be fooled into an inappropriate analysis just because others, in similar circumstances, have done one in the past!
- Take an appropriate transformation of the raw data so that the transformed data satisfy the assumptions of the proposed analysis (Topic 9);
- If feasible, perform a **non-parametric analysis** (Topic 17) that does not make any assumption about the distribution of the data (e.g. Normality).

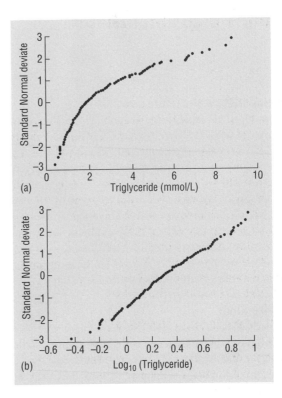

Fig. 32.1 (a) Normal plot of untransformed triglyceride levels described in Topic 19. These are skewed and the resulting Normal plot shows a distinct curve. (b) Normal plot of log triglyceride levels. The approximately straight line indicates that the log transformation has been successful at removing the skewness in the data.

Example

Consider the unpaired t-test example of Topic 21. A total of 98 school age children were randomly assigned to receive either inhaled beclomethasone dipropionate or a placebo to determine their effects on wheezing. We used the unpaired t-test to compare the mean forced expiratory volume (FEV1) in each group over the 6 months, but need assurance that the underlying assumptions (Normality and constant variance) are satisfied. The stem-and-leaf plots in Fig. 4.2 show that the data in each group are approximately Normally distributed. We performed the **F-test** to investigate the assumption of constant variance in the two groups.

1 H_0: the variance of FEV1 measurements in the population of school age children is the same in the two treatment groups

 H_1: the variance of FEV1 measurements in the population of school age children is not the same in two treatment groups.

2 Treated group: sample size, $n_1 = 50$, standard deviation, $s_1 = 0.291$
Placebo group: sample size, $n_2 = 48$, standard deviation, $s_2 = 0.251$

3 The test statistic, $F = \dfrac{s_1^2}{s_2^2} = \dfrac{0.29^2}{0.25^2} = \dfrac{0.0841}{0.0625} = 1.336$

which follows an F-distribution with $50 - 1 = 49$ and $48 - 1 = 47$ df in the numerator and denominator, respectively.

4 We refer $F = 1.34$ to Appendix A5 for a two-sided test at the 5% level of significance. Because Appendix A5 is restricted to entries of 25 and infinity df in the numerator, and 30 and 50 df in the denominator, we have to interpolate (Topic 21). The required tabulated value at the 5% level of significance lies between 1.57 and 2.12; thus $P > 0.05$ because 1.34 is less than the minimum of these values.

5 There is insufficient evidence to reject the null hypothesis that the variances are equal. It is reasonable to use the unpaired t-test, which assumes Normality and homogeneity of variance, to compare the mean FEV1 values in the two groups.

33 Sample size calculations

The importance of sample size

The number of patients in a study is usually restricted because of ethical, cost and time considerations. If our sample size is too small, however, we may not be able to detect an important existing effect [i.e. the power (Topic 18) of the test will be inadequate], and we shall have wasted all our resources. We therefore have to optimize the sample size, striking a balance between sample size and the factors (such as power, the size of the treatment effect and the significance level) that affect it. Unfortunately, in order to calculate the sample size required, we have to have some idea of the results we expect in the study.

Requirements

We shall explain how to calculate the optimal sample size in simple situations; often more complex designs can be simplified for the purpose of calculating the sample size. If our investigation involves a number of tests, we focus on the most important or evaluate the sample size required for each and choose the largest.

To calculate sample size, we need to specify the following quantities, *at the design stage of the investigation*.
- **Power** (Topic 18)—the chance of detecting, as statistically significant, a specified effect if it exists. We usually choose the power to equal 70–80% or more.
- **Significance level**, α (Topic 17)—the cut-off level below which we will reject the null hypothesis, i.e. it is the maximum probability of incorrectly concluding that there is an effect. We usually fix this as 0.05, or occasionally, 0.01, and reject the null hypothesis if the *P*-value is less than this value.
- **Variability** of the observations, e.g. the standard deviation, if we have a numerical variable.
- **Smallest effect of interest**—the magnitude of the effect that is clinically important and that we do not want to overlook. This is often a *difference* (e.g. difference in means or proportions). Sometimes it is expressed as a multiple of the standard deviation of the observations (the **standardized difference**).

It is relatively simple to choose the power and significance level of the test that suits the particular requirements of our study. Given a particular clinical scenario, it is possible to specify the effect we regard as clinically important. The real difficulty lies in providing an estimate of the variation in a numerical variable before we have collected the data.

Methodology

We can calculate sample size in a number of ways, each of which requires essentially the same information (described in Requirements) in order to proceed.
- **General formulae**—these can be complex.
- **Quick formulae**—these exist for particular power values and significance levels for some hypothesis tests (e.g. Lehr's formulae[1], see below).
- **Special tables**[2]—these exist for particular hypothesis tests, e.g. unpaired *t*-test or Chi-squared test.
- **Altman's nomogram**—this is an easy-to-use diagram that is appropriate for various tests. Details are given in the next section.
- **Computer software**—this has the advantage that results can be presented graphically or in tables to show the consequence of changing the factors (e.g. power, size of effect) on the required sample size.

Altman's nomogram
Notation

We show in Table 33.1 the notation for using Altman's nomogram to estimate the sample size of two *equally sized* groups of observations for three frequently used hypothesis tests of means and proportions.

Method

For each test, we calculate the standardized difference and join its value on the left hand axis of the nomogram (Appendix B) to the power we have specified on the right-hand vertical axis. The required sample size is indicated at the point at which the resulting line and sample size axis meet.

Note that we can also use the nomogram to evaluate the power of a hypothesis test for a given sample size. Occasionally, this is useful if we wish to know, retrospectively, whether we can attribute lack of significance in a hypothesis test to an inadequately sized sample. Remember, also, that a wide confidence interval for the effect of interest indicates poor power (Topic 11).

Quick formulae

For the unpaired *t*-test and Chi-squared test, we can use Lehr's formula[1] for calculating the sample size for a power

[1] Lehr, R. (1992) Sixteen s squared over d squared: a relation for crude sample size estimates. *Statistics in Medicine*, **11**, 1099–1102.
[2] Machin, D. & Campbell, M.J. (1995) *Statistical Tables for the Design of Clinical Trials*, 2nd edn. Blackwell Scientific Publications, Oxford.

of 80% and a two-sided significance level of 0.05. The required sample size in each group is:

$$\frac{16}{(Standardized\ difference)^2}$$

If the standardized difference is small, this overestimates the sample size. Note that a numerator of 21 (instead of 16) relates to a power of 90%.

Power statement

It is often essential and always useful to include a power statement in a study protocol or in the methods section of a paper to show that careful thought has been given to sample size at the design stage of the investigation. A typical statement might be '84 patients in each group were required to have a 90% chance of detecting a difference in means of 2.5 days (SD = 5 days) at the 5% level of significance using the unpaired t-test' (see Example 1).

Table 33.1 Information for using Altman's nomogram.

Hypothesis test	Standardized difference	Explanation of N	Terminology
Unpaired t-test (Topic 21)	$\dfrac{\delta}{\sigma}$	$N/2$ observations in each group	δ: the smallest difference in means that is clinically important. σ: the assumed equal standard deviation of the observations in each of the two groups. You can estimate it using results from a similar study conducted previously or from published information. Alternatively, you could perform a pilot study to estimate it. Another approach is to express δ as a multiple of the standard deviation (e.g. the ability to detect a difference of two standard deviations).
Paired t-test (Topic 20)	$\dfrac{2\delta}{\sigma_d}$	N pairs of observations	δ: the smallest mean difference that is clinically important. σ_d: the standard deviation of the *differences* in response, usually estimated from a pilot study.
Chi-squared test (Topic 24)	$\dfrac{p_1 - p_2}{\sqrt{\bar{p}(1-\bar{p})}}$	$N/2$ observations in each group	$p_1 - p_2$: the smallest difference in the proportions of 'success' in the two groups that is clinically important. One of these proportions is often known, and the relevant difference evaluated by considering what value the other proportion must take in order to constitute a noteworthy change. $\bar{p} = \dfrac{p_1 + p_2}{2}$

Example 1
Comparing means in independent groups using the unpaired t-test

Objective—to examine the effectiveness of aciclovir suspension (15 mg/kg) for treating 1–7-year-old children with herpetic gingivostomatitis lasting less than 72 h.

Design—randomized, double-blind placebo-controlled trial with 'treatment' administered five times a day for 7 days.

Main outcome measure for determining sample size—duration of oral lesions.

Sample size question—how many children are required to have a 90% power of detecting a 2.5 day difference in duration of oral lesions between the two groups at the 5% level of significance? The authors assume that the standard deviation of duration of oral lesions is approximately 5 days.

continued

Using the nomogram:

$\delta = 2.5$ days and $\sigma = 5$ days. Thus standardized difference equals $\dfrac{\delta}{\sigma} = \dfrac{2.5}{5} = 0.50$

The line connecting a standardized difference of 0.50 and a power of 90% cuts the sample size axis at approximately 160. Therefore, about 80 children are required in each group (*note*: if δ were increased to 3 days, the standardized difference equals 0.6 and the required sample size would decrease to approximately 118 in total, i.e. 59 in each group).

Quick formula:

If the power is 90%, the required sample size in each group is: $\dfrac{21}{(standardized\ difference\ )^2} = \dfrac{21}{(0.50)^2} = 84.$

Amir, J., Haral, L., Smettana, Z., Varsano, I. (1977) Treatment of herpes simplex gingivostomatitis with aciclovir in children: a randomised double-blind placebo-controlled study. *British Medical Journal*, **314**, 1800–1803.

Example 2

Comparing two proportions in independent groups using the Chi-squared test

Objective—to compare the effectiveness of corticosteroid injections with physiotherapy for the treatment of painful stiff shoulder.

Design—Randomized controlled trial (RCT) in which patients are randomly allocated to 6 weeks of treatment, these comprising either a maximum of three injections or twelve 30 min sessions of physiotherapy for each patient.

Main outcome measure for determining sample size—treatment is regarded as a success after 7 weeks if the patient rates him/herself as having made a complete recovery or as having much improvement (on a six-point Likert scale).

Sample size question—how many patients are required in order to have an 80% power of detecting a clinically important difference in success rates of 25% between the two groups at the 5% level of significance? The authors assume a success rate of 40% in the group having the least successful treatment.

Using the nomogram:

$p_1 = 0.40$ and $p_2 = 0.65$, so $\bar{p} = \dfrac{0.40 + 0.65}{2} = 0.525$

Therefore, standardized difference

$= \dfrac{p_1 - p_2}{\sqrt{\bar{p}(1 - \bar{p})}} = \dfrac{0.25}{\sqrt{0.525 \times 0.475}} = 0.50$

The line connecting a standardized difference of 0.50 and a power of 80% cuts the sample size axis at 120. Therefore approximately 60 patients are required in each group (*note*: if the power were increased to 85%, the required sample size would increase to approximately 140 in total, i.e. 70 patients would be required in each group).

Quick formula:

If the power is 80%, the required sample size in each group is: $\dfrac{16}{(standardized\ difference\ )^2} = \dfrac{16}{(0.50)^2} = 64.$

van der Windt, D.A.W.M., Koes, B.W., Devillé, W., de Jong, B.A., Bouter, M. (1998) Effectiveness of corticosteroid injections with physiotherapy for treatment of painful shoulder in primary care: randomised trial. *British Medical Journal*, **317**, 1292–1296.

Figures 18.1 and 18.2 show power curves for these examples.

34 Presenting results

Introduction

An essential facet of statistics is the ability to summarize the important features of the analysis. We must know what to include and how to display our results in a manner that enables others to obtain relevant and important information easily and draw correct conclusions. This topic describes the key features of presentation.

Numerical results

- Give figures only to the degree of accuracy that is appropriate (as a guideline, one significant figure more than the raw data). If analysing the data by hand, only round up or down at the end of the calculations.
- Give the number of items on which any summary measure (e.g. a percentage) is based.
- Describe any outliers and explain how they are handled (Topic 3).
- Include the units of measurement.
- When interest is focused on a parameter (e.g. the mean, regression coefficient), always indicate the precision of its estimate. We recommend using a confidence interval for this but the standard error is also acceptable. *Avoid* using the ± symbol, as in mean ± SEM (Topic 10), because by adding and subtracting the SEM, we create a 67% confidence interval that can be misleading for those used to 95% confidence intervals. It is better to show the standard error in brackets after the parameter estimate [e.g. mean = 16.6 g (SEM 0.5 g)].
- When interest is focused on the distribution of observations, always indicate a measure of the 'spread' of the data. The range of values that excludes outliers (typically, the range of values containing the central 95% of the observations—Topic 6) is a useful descriptor. If the data are Normally distributed, this range is approximated by the sample mean ± 1.96 × standard deviation (Topic 7). You can quote the mean and the standard deviation [e.g. mean = 35.9 mm (SD 2.8 mm)] instead but this leaves the reader to evaluate the range.

Tables

- Do not give too much information in a table.
- Include a concise, informative, and unambiguous title.
- Label each row and column.
- Remember that it is easier to scan information down columns rather than across rows.

Diagrams

- Keep a diagram simple and avoid unnecessary frills (e.g. making a pie chart three-dimensional).
- Include a concise, informative, and unambiguous title.

- Label all axes, segments, and bars, and explain the meaning of symbols.
- Avoid distorting results by exaggerating the scale on an axis.
- Indicate where two or more observations lie in the same position on a scatter diagram, e.g. by using a different symbol.
- Ensure that all the relevant information is contained in the diagram (e.g. link paired observations).

Presenting results in a paper

When presenting results in a paper, we should ensure that the paper contains enough information for the reader to understand what has been done. He/she should be able to reproduce the results, given the appropriate computer package and data. All aspects of the design of the study and the statistical methodology must be fully described.

Results of a hypothesis test

- Include a relevant diagram, if appropriate.
- Indicate the hypotheses of interest.
- Name the test and state whether it is one- or two-tailed.
- Justify the assumptions (if any) underlying the test (e.g. Normality, constant variance), and describe any transformations (Topic 9) required to meet these assumptions (e.g. taking logarithms).
- Specify the observed value of the test statistic, its distribution (and degrees of freedom, if relevant), and, if possible, the *exact* P-value (e.g. $P = 0.03$) rather than an interval estimate of it (e.g. $0.01 < P < 0.05$) or a star system (e.g. *, **, *** for increasing levels of significance). Avoid writing 'n.s.' when $P > 0.05$; an exact P-value is preferable even when the result is non-significant.
- Include an estimate of the *relevant* effect of interest (e.g. the difference in means for the two-sample t-test, or the mean difference for the paired t-test) with a confidence interval (preferably) or standard error.
- Draw conclusions from the results (e.g. reject the null hypothesis), interpret any confidence interval and explain their implications.

Results of a regression analysis

Here we include simple (Topics 27 and 28) and multiple linear regression (Topic 29), logistic regression (Topic 30), and proportional hazards regression (Topic 41). Full details of these analyses are explained in the associated topics.

- Include relevant diagrams (e.g. a scatter plot with the fitted line for simple regression).
- Clearly state which is the dependent variable and which is (are) the explanatory variable(s).

- Justify underlying assumptions.
- Describe any transformations, and explain their purpose.
- Where appropriate, describe the possible numerical values taken by any categorical variable (e.g. male = 0, female = 1), how dummy variables were created, and the units of continuous variables.
- Give an indication of the goodness-of-fit of the model (e.g. quote R^2).
- If appropriate (e.g. in multiple regression), give the results of the overall F-test from the ANOVA table.
- Provide estimates of *all* the coefficients in the model (including those which are not significant) together with the confidence intervals for the coefficients or standard errors of their estimates. In logistic regression (Topic 30) and proportional hazards regression (Topic 41), convert the coefficients to estimated odds ratios or relative hazards (with confidence intervals). Interpret the relevant coefficients.

- Show the results of the hypothesis tests on the coefficients (i.e. include the test statistics and the P-values). Draw appropriate conclusions from these tests.

Complex analyses

There are no simple rules for the presentation of the more complex forms of statistical analysis. Be sure to describe the design of the study fully (e.g. the factors in the analysis of variance and whether there is a hierarchical arrangement), and include a validation of underlying assumptions, relevant descriptive statistics (with confidence intervals), test statistics and P-values. A brief description of what the analysis is doing helps the uninitiated; this should be accompanied by a reference for further details. Specify which computer package has been used.

Example

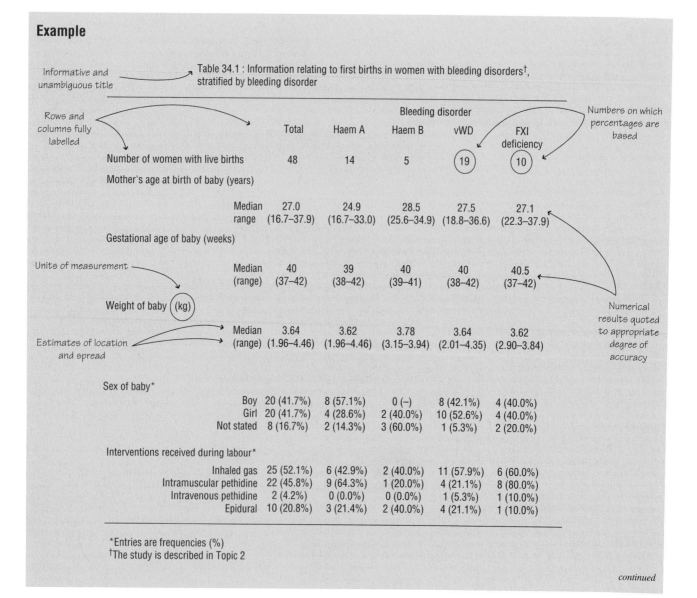

Table 34.1 : Information relating to first births in women with bleeding disorders[†], stratified by bleeding disorder

		Total	Haem A	Haem B	vWD	FXI deficiency
Number of women with live births		48	14	5	19	10
Mother's age at birth of baby (years)						
	Median	27.0	24.9	28.5	27.5	27.1
	range	(16.7–37.9)	(16.7–33.0)	(25.6–34.9)	(18.8–36.6)	(22.3–37.9)
Gestational age of baby (weeks)						
	Median	40	39	40	40	40.5
	(range)	(37–42)	(38–42)	(39–41)	(38–42)	(37–42)
Weight of baby (kg)						
	Median	3.64	3.62	3.78	3.64	3.62
	(range)	(1.96–4.46)	(1.96–4.46)	(3.15–3.94)	(2.01–4.35)	(2.90–3.84)
Sex of baby*						
	Boy	20 (41.7%)	8 (57.1%)	0 (–)	8 (42.1%)	4 (40.0%)
	Girl	20 (41.7%)	4 (28.6%)	2 (40.0%)	10 (52.6%)	4 (40.0%)
	Not stated	8 (16.7%)	2 (14.3%)	3 (60.0%)	1 (5.3%)	2 (20.0%)
Interventions received during labour*						
	Inhaled gas	25 (52.1%)	6 (42.9%)	2 (40.0%)	11 (57.9%)	6 (60.0%)
	Intramuscular pethidine	22 (45.8%)	9 (64.3%)	1 (20.0%)	4 (21.1%)	8 (80.0%)
	Intravenous pethidine	2 (4.2%)	0 (0.0%)	0 (0.0%)	1 (5.3%)	1 (10.0%)
	Epidural	10 (20.8%)	3 (21.4%)	2 (40.0%)	4 (21.1%)	1 (10.0%)

*Entries are frequencies (%)
[†]The study is described in Topic 2

Informative and unambiguous title · *Rows and columns fully labelled* · *Numbers on which percentages are based* · *Units of measurement* · *Numerical results quoted to appropriate degree of accuracy* · *Estimates of location and spread*

continued

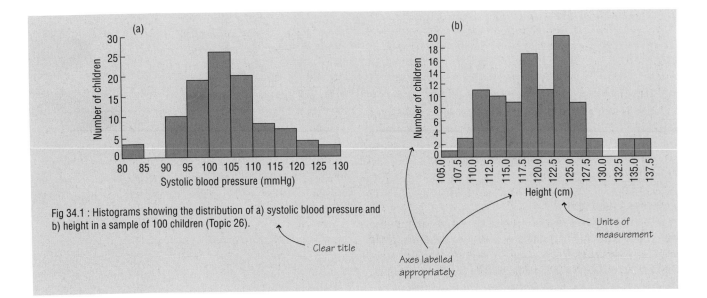

Fig 34.1 : Histograms showing the distribution of a) systolic blood pressure and b) height in a sample of 100 children (Topic 26).

Clear title

Axes labelled appropriately

Units of measurement

35 Diagnostic tools

An individual's health is often characterized by a number of numerical or categorical measures. We can use **reference intervals** (Topics 6 and 7) and **diagnostic tests** to determine whether the measurement seen in an individual is likely to be the consequence of undiagnosed illness or may be indicative of disease.

Reference intervals

A **reference interval** (often referred to as a **normal range**) for a single numerical variable, calculated from a very large sample, provides a range of values that are typically seen in healthy individuals. If an individual's value is above the upper limit, or below the lower limit, we consider it to be unusually high (or low) relative to healthy individuals.

Calculating reference intervals

Two approaches can be taken.
• We make the assumption that the data are Normally distributed. Approximately 95% of the data values lie within 1.96 standard deviations of the mean (Topic 7). We use our data to calculate these two limits (mean ± 1.96 standard deviations).
• An alternative approach, which does not make any assumptions about the distribution of the measurement, is to use a central range which encompasses 95% of the data values (Topic 6). We put our values in order of magnitude and use the 2.5th and 97.5th percentiles as our limits.

The effect of other factors on reference intervals

Sometimes the values of a numerical variable depend on other factors, such as age or sex. It is important to interpret a particular value only after considering these other factors. For example, we generate reference intervals for systolic blood pressure separately for men and women.

Diagnostic tests

The **gold-standard test** that provides a definitive diagnosis of a particular condition may sometimes be impractical. We would like a simple test, depending on the presence or absence of some marker, which provides an accurate guide to whether or not the patient has the condition.

We take a group of individuals whose true disease status is known from the gold standard test. We can draw up the 2×2 table of frequencies (Table 35.1):

Table 35.1 Table of frequencies.

Test result	Gold standard test		
	Disease	No disease	Total
Positive	a	b	$a+b$
Negative	c	d	$c+d$
Total	$a+c$	$b+d$	$n=a+b+c+d$

Of the n individuals studied, $a + c$ individuals have the disease. The **prevalence** (Topic 12) of the disease in this sample is $= \dfrac{(a+c)}{n}$.

Of the $a + c$ individuals who have the disease, a have positive test results (**true positives**) and c have negative test results (**false negatives**). Of the $b + d$ individuals who do not have the disease, d have negative test results (**true negatives**) and b have positive test results (**false positives**).

Assessing reliability: sensitivity and specificity

Sensitivity = proportion of individuals with the disease who are correctly identified by the test

$$= \frac{a}{(a+c)}$$

Specificity = proportion of individuals without the disease who are correctly identified by the test

$$= \frac{d}{(b+d)}$$

These are usually expressed as percentages. As with all estimates, we should calculate confidence intervals for these measures (Topic 11).

We would like to have a sensitivity and specificity that are both as close to 1 (or 100%) as possible. However, in practice, we may gain sensitivity at the expense of specificity, and vice versa. Whether we aim for a high sensitivity or high specificity depends on the condition we are trying to detect, along with the implications for the patient and/or the population of either a false negative or false positive test result. For conditions that are easily treatable, we prefer a high sensitivity; for those that are serious and untreatable, we prefer a high specificity in order to avoid making a false positive diagnosis.

Predictive values

Positive predictive value = proportion of individuals with a positive test result who have the disease

$$= \frac{a}{(a+b)}$$

Negative predictive value = proportion of individuals with a negative test result who do not have the disease

$$= \frac{d}{(c+d)}$$

We calculate confidence intervals for these predictive values, often expressed as percentages, using the methods described in Topic 11.

These predictive values provide information about how likely it is that the individual has or does not have the disease, given his/her test result. Predictive values are dependent on the prevalence of the disease in the population being studied. In populations where the disease is common, the positive predictive value will be much higher than in populations where the disease is rare. The converse is true for negative predictive values.

The use of a cut-off value

Sometimes we wish to make a diagnosis on the basis of a continuous measurement. Often there is no threshold above (or below) which disease definitely occurs. In these situations, we need to define a cut-off value ourselves, above (or below) which we believe an individual has a very high chance of having the disease.

A useful approach is to use the upper (or lower) limit of the reference interval. We can evaluate this cut-off value by calculating its associated sensitivity, specificity and predictive values. If we choose a different cut-off, these values may change as we become more or less stringent. We choose the cut-off to optimize these measures as desired.

Receiver operating characteristic curves

These provide a way of assessing whether a particular type of test provides useful information, and can be used to compare two different tests, and to select an optimal cut-off value for a test.

For a given test, we consider all cut-off points that give a unique pair of values for sensitivity and specificity, and plot the *sensitivity* against 1 *minus the specificity* (thus comparing the probabilities of a positive test result in those with and without disease) and connect these points by lines (Fig. 35.1).

The receiver operating characteristic (ROC) curve for a test that has some use will lie to the left of the diagonal of the graph. Two or more tests can be compared by considering the area under each curve—the test with the greater area is better. Depending on the implications of false positive and false negative results, and the prevalence of the condition, we can choose the optimal cut-off value for a test from this graph.

Is a test useful?

The **likelihood ratio** (LR) for a positive result is the ratio of the chance of a positive result if the patient has the disease to the chance of a positive result if he/she does not have the disease. Likelihood ratios can also be generated for negative test results. For example, a LR of 2 for a positive result indicates that a positive result is twice as likely to occur in an individual with disease than in one without it. A high likelihood ratio for a positive result suggests that the test provides useful information, as does a likelihood ratio close to zero for a negative result.

It can be shown that:

LR for a positive result $= \dfrac{Sensitivity}{(1 - specificity)}$

We discuss the LR further in Topic 42.

Example

Cytomegalovirus (CMV) is a common viral infection to which approximately 50% of individuals are exposed during childhood. Although infection with the virus does not usually lead to any major problems, individuals who have been infected with CMV in the past may suffer serious disease after certain transplant procedures, such as bone marrow transplantation, if their virus is either reactivated or if they are re-infected by their donors. It is thought that the amount of detectable virus in their blood after transplantation (the viral load) may predict which individuals will get severe disease. In order to study this hypothesis, CMV viral load was measured in a group of 49 bone marrow transplant recipients. Fifteen of the 49 patients developed severe disease during follow-up. Viral load values in all patients ranged from 2.7 $\log_{10}$ genomes/mL to 6.0 $\log_{10}$ genomes/mL. As a starting point, a value in excess of 4.5 $\log_{10}$ genomes/mL was considered an indication of the possible future development of disease. The table of frequencies below shows the results

	Severe disease		
Viral load ($\log_{10}$ genomes/mL)	Yes	No	Total
>4.5	7	6	13
≤4.5	8	28	36
Total	15	34	49

Sensitivity $= 7/15 \times 100\% = 47\%$ (95% CI 22% to 72%)

Specificity $= 28/34 \times 100\% = 82\%$ (95% CI 69% to 95%)

Positive predictive value $= 7/13 \times 100\% = 54\%$ (95% CI 27% to 81%)

Negative predictive value $= 28/36 \times 100\% = 78\%$ (95% CI 65% to 92%)

Likelihood ratio for positive result $= 0.47/(1-0.82) = 2.6$ (95% CI 1.1% to 6.5, obtained from computer output)

obtained; the box contains calculations of measures of interest.

Therefore, for this cut-off value, we have a relatively high specificity and a moderate sensitivity. The LR of 2.6 indicates that this test is useful, in that a viral load >4.5 $\log_{10}$ genomes/mL is more than twice as likely in an individual with severe disease than in one without severe disease. However, in order to investigate other cut-off values, a ROC curve was plotted (Fig. 35.1). The plotted line falls just to the left of the diagonal of the graph. For this example, the most useful cut-off value (5.0 $\log_{10}$ genomes/mL) is that which gives a sensitivity of 40% and a specificity of 97%; then the LR equals 13.3.

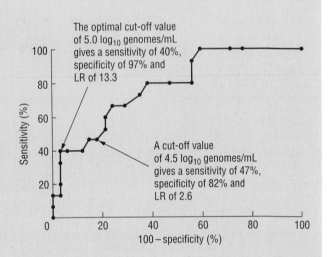

Fig. 35.1 Receiver operating characteristic (ROC) curve, indicating the results from two possible cut-off values, the optimal one and that used in the diagnostic test.

Data kindly provided by Dr V.C. Emery and Dr D. Gor, Department of Virology, Royal Free and University College Medical School, Royal Free Campus, London, UK.

36 Assessing agreement

Introduction

There are many occasions on which we wish to compare results that should concur. In particular, we may want to assess and, if possible, quantify the following two types of agreement.
- **Reproducibility (method/observer agreement)**. Do two techniques used to measure a particular variable, in otherwise identical circumstances, produce the same result? Do two or more observers using the same method of measurement obtain the same results?
- **Repeatability**. Does a single observer obtain the same results when he/she takes repeated measurements in identical circumstances?

Both reproducibility and repeatability can be approached in the same way. In each case, the method of analysis depends on whether the variable is **categorical** (e.g. poor/average/good) or **numerical** (e.g. systolic blood pressure). For simplicity, we shall restrict the problem to that of comparing only **two** sets of paired results (e.g. two methods/two observers/duplicate measurements).

Categorical variables

Suppose two observers assess the same patients for disease severity using a categorical scale of measurement, and we wish to evaluate the extent to which they agree. We present the results in a two-way contingency table of frequencies with the rows and columns indicating the categories of response for each observer. Table 36.1 is an example, showing the results of two observers' assessments of the condition of tooth surfaces. The frequencies with which the observers agree are shown along the **diagonal** of the table. We calculate the corresponding frequencies that would be **expected** if the categorizations were made at random in the same way as we calculated expected frequencies in the Chi-squared test of association (Topic 24); i.e. each expected frequency is the product of the relevant row and column totals divided by the overall total. Then we measure agreement by:

$$Cohen's\ kappa,\ \kappa = \frac{\left(\dfrac{O_d}{m} - \dfrac{E_d}{m}\right)}{\left(1 - \dfrac{E_d}{m}\right)}$$

which represents the chance corrected proportional agreement, where:
- m is the total observed frequency (e.g. total number of patients);
- O_d is the sum of observed frequencies *along the diagonal*;

- E_d is the sum of expected frequencies *along the diagonal*;
- 1 in the denominator represents maximum agreement.

$\kappa = 1$ implies perfect agreement and $\kappa = 0$ suggests that the agreement is no better than that which would be obtained by chance. There are no objective criteria for judging intermediate values. However, kappa is often judged as providing agreement[1] which is:

- poor if $\kappa \leq 0.20$;
- fair if $0.21 \leq \kappa \leq 0.40$;
- moderate if $0.41 \leq \kappa \leq 0.60$;
- substantial if $0.61 \leq \kappa \leq 0.80$;
- good if $\kappa > 0.80$.

Note that kappa is dependent both on the number of categories (i.e. its value is greater if there are fewer categories) and the prevalence of the condition, so care must be taken when comparing kappas from different studies. For ordinal data, we can also calculate a **weighted kappa**[2], which takes into account the extent to which the observers **disagree** (the non-diagonal frequencies) as well as the frequencies of agreement (along the diagonal).

Numerical variables

Suppose an observer takes duplicate measurements of a numerical variable on n individuals (just replace the word 'repeatability' by 'reproducibility' if considering the similar problem of method agreement).
- If the average difference (e.g. the true mean difference, estimated by $\bar{d}$) is zero (as assessed by the paired t-test, sign test or signed ranks test—Topics 19 and 20) then we can infer that there is no **bias** in the results. This implies that, *on average*, the duplicate readings agree.
- The estimated standard deviation of the differences (s_d) provides a measure of agreement that can be used as a comparative tool. However, it is more usual to calculate the **British Standards Institution repeatability coefficient** $= 2s_d$. This indicates the maximum difference that is likely to occur between two measurements if there is no bias. Assuming a Normal distribution of differences, we expect approximately 95% of the differences in the population to lie between $\bar{d} \pm 2s_d$. The upper and lower limits of this interval are called the **limits of agreement**; from them, we can

[1] Landis, J.R. & Koch, G.G. (1977) The measurement of observer agreement for categorical data. *Biometrics*, **33**, 159–174.
[2] Cohen, J. (1968) Weighted kappa: nominal scale agreement with provision for scale disagreement or partial credit. *Psychological Bulletin*, **70**, 213–220.

decide (subjectively) whether the agreement between pairs of readings in a given situation is acceptable.

Precautions

• It makes no sense to calculate a single measure of repeatability if the extent to which the observations in a pair disagree depends on the magnitude of the measurement. We can check this by determining both the mean of and the difference between each pair of readings, and plotting the n differences against their corresponding means[3] (Fig. 36.1). If there is no relationship, then we should observe a random scatter of points (evenly distributed above and below zero if no bias is present). If, however, we observe a funnel effect, with the variation in the differences being greater (say) for larger mean values, then we must reassess the problem. We may be able to find an appropriate transformation of the raw data (Topic 9), so that when we repeat the process on the transformed observations, the required condition is satisfied. We can also use the plot to detect outliers (Topic 3).

• Be wary of producing a scatter diagram with the results from the first occasion plotted against those from the second occasion (or the data from one method/observer plotted against the other), and calculating the correlation coefficient (Topic 26). We are not really interested in whether the points lie on a straight line; we want to know whether they conform to the 45° line, i.e. the line of equality. This will not be established by a hypothesis test of the null hypothesis that the true correlation coefficient is zero. Furthermore, bear in mind the fact that it is possible to increase the magnitude of the correlation coefficient by increasing the range of values of the measurements.

More complex situations

Sometimes you may come across more complex problems when assessing agreement. For example, there may be more than two replicates, or more than two observers, or each of a number of observers may have replicate observations. You can find details of the analysis of such problems in Streiner and Norman[4].

Example 1

Assessing agreement — categorical variable

Two observers, an experienced dentist and a dental student, assessed the condition of 2104 tooth surfaces in school-aged children. Every surface was coded as '0' (sound), '1' (with at least one 'small' cavity), '2' (with at least one 'big' cavity) or '3' (with at least one filling, with or without cavities) by each individual. The observed frequencies are shown in Table 36.1. The bold figures along the diagonal show the observed frequencies of agreement; the corresponding expected frequencies are in brackets. We calculated **Cohen's Kappa** to assess the agreement between the two observers.

We estimate Cohen's kappa as:

$$\kappa = \frac{\left(\dfrac{1785 + 154 + 20 + 14}{2104}\right) - \left(\dfrac{1602.1 + 21.3 + 0.5 + 0.2}{2104}\right)}{1 - \left(\dfrac{1602.1 + 21.3 + 0.5 + 0.2}{2104}\right)}$$

$$= \frac{0.9377 - 0.7719}{1 - 0.7719} = 0.73$$

There appears to be substantial agreement between the student and the experienced dentist in the coding of the children's tooth surfaces.

Table 36.1 Observed (and expected) frequencies of tooth surface assessments.

		Dental student				
	Code	0	1	2	3	Total
Dentist	0	**1785** (1602.1)	46	0	7	1838
	1	46	**154** (21.3)	18	5	223
	2	0	0	**20** (0.5)	0	25
	3	3	1	0	**14** (0.2)	18
	Total	1834	201	43	26	2104

Data kindly provided by Dr R.D. Holt, Department of Transcultural Oral Health, Eastman Dental Institute for Oral Health Care Sciences, University College London, London, UK.

---

[3] Bland, J.M. & Altman, D.G. (1986) Statistical methods for assessing agreement between two pairs of clinical measurement. *Lancet*, **i**, 307–310.

[4] Streiner, G.L. & Norman, D.R. (1990) *Health Measurement Scales: A Practical Guide to their Development and Use.* Oxford University Press, Oxford.

Example 2

Assessing agreement—numerical variable

The Rosenberg self-esteem index is used to judge a patient's evaluation of his or her own self-esteem. The maximum value of the index (an indication of high self-esteem) for a person is 50, comprising the sum of the individual values from 10 questions, each scored from zero to five. Part of a study that examined the effectiveness of a particular type of surgery for facial deformity examined the change in a patient's psychological profile by comparing the values of the Rosenberg index in the patient before and after surgery. The investigators were concerned about the extent to which the Rosenberg score would be reliable for a set of patients, and decided to assess the **repeatability** of the measure on the first 25 patients requesting treatment for facial deformity. They obtained a value for the Rosenberg index when the patient initially presented at the clinic and then asked the patient for a second assessment 4 weeks later. The results are shown in Table 36.2.

The differences (first value—second value) can be shown to be approximately Normally distributed; they have a mean, $\bar{d} = 0.56$ and standard deviation, $s_d = 1.83$. The test statistic for the paired t-test is equal to 1.53 (degrees of freedom = 24), giving $P = 0.14$. This non-significant result indicates that there is no evidence of any bias.

The British Standards Institution repeatability coefficient is $2s_d = 2 \times 1.83 = 3.7$. Approximately 95% of the differences in the population of such patients would be expected to lie between $\bar{d} \pm 2s_d$, i.e. between −3.1 and 4.3. These limits are indicated in Fig. 36.1, which shows that the differences are randomly scattered around a mean of approximately zero. On the basis of these results, the investigators felt that the Rosenberg index was reliable, and used it to evaluate the patients' perceptions of the effectiveness of the facial surgery.

Table 36.2 The pre-treatment values (1st and 2nd) of the Rosenberg index obtained on 25 patients.

1st	2nd	1st	2nd	1st	2nd	1st	2nd	1st	2nd
30	27	41	39	37	39	43	43	21	20
39	41	41	41	42	42	40	39	41	39
50	49	60	49	46	44	31	30	29	28
45	42	38	40	49	48	45	46	26	27
25	28	41	39	21	23	46	42	32	30

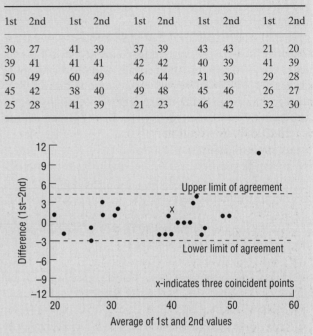

Fig. 36.1 Difference between first and second Rosenberg self-esteem values plotted against their average for 25 patients.

Adapted from: Cunningham, S.J., Hunt, N.P., Feinnman, C. (1996) Perceptions of outcome following orthognathic surgery. *British Journal of Oral and Maxillofacial Surgery*, **34**, 210–213.

37 Evidence-based medicine

Sackett et al.[1] describe **evidence-based medicine (EBM)** as 'the conscientious, explicit and judicious use of current best evidence in making decisions about the care of individual patients'. To practice EBM, you must be able to locate the research relevant to the care of your patients, and judge its quality. Only then can you think about applying the findings in clinical practice.

Sackett et al. suggest the following approach to EBM. For convenience, we have phrased the third and fourth points below in terms of clinical trials (Topic 14) and observational studies (Topics 15 and 16), but they can be modified to suit other forms of investigations (e.g. diagnostic tests, Topic 35).

1   Formulate the problem

You must decide what is of interest to you—how you define the patient population, which intervention (e.g. treatment) or comparison is relevant, and what outcome you are looking at (e.g. reduced mortality).

2   Locate the relevant information (e.g. on diagnosis, prognosis or therapy)

Often the relevant information will be found in published papers, but you should also consider other possibilities, such as conference abstracts. You must know what databases (e.g. Medline) and other sources of evidence are available, how they are organized, which search terms to use, and how to operate the searching software.

3   Critically appraise the methods in order to assess the validity (closeness to the truth) of the evidence

The following questions should be asked.
- Have all **important** *outcomes* been considered?
- Was the study conducted using an **appropriate spectrum of patients**?
- Do the results make **biological sense**?
- Was the study designed to eliminate **bias**? For example, in a clinical trial, was the study **controlled**, was **randomization** used in the assignment of patients, was the assessment of response '**blind**', were any patients lost to follow-up, were the groups treated in similar fashion, aside from the fact that they received different treatments, and was an '**intention-to-treat**' analysis performed?
- Are the statistical methods appropriate (e.g. have underlying assumptions been verified; have dependencies in the data (e.g. pairing) been taken into account in the analysis)?

[1] Sackett, D.L., Richardson, W.S., Rosenberg, W., Haynes, R.B. (1997) *Evidence-based Medicine: How to Practice and Teach EBM*. Churchill-Livingstone, London.

4   Extract the most useful results and determine whether they are important

Extracting the most useful results

You should ask the following questions:

(a) What is the **main outcome variable** (i.e. that which relates to the major objective)?

(b) How **large** is the **effect of interest**, expressed in terms of the main outcome variable? If this variable is:

- **Binary** (e.g. died/survived)
  (i) What are the rates of occurrence of this event (e.g. death) in the (two) comparison groups?
  (ii) The effect of interest may be the difference in rates (the absolute reduction in risk) or the ratio of rates (the relative risk or odds ratio)—what is its magnitude?

- **Numerical** (e.g. systolic blood pressure)
  (i) What is the mean (or median) value of the variable in each of the comparison groups?
  (ii) What is the effect of interest, i.e. the difference in means (medians)?

(c) How **precise** is the **effect of interest**? Ideally, the research being scrutinized should include the confidence interval for the true effect (a wide confidence interval is an indication of poor precision). Is this confidence interval quoted? If not, is sufficient information (e.g. the standard error of the effect of interest) provided so that the confidence interval can be determined?

Deciding whether the results are important

- Consider the **confidence interval** for the effect of interest (e.g. the difference in treatment means):
  (i) Would you regard the observed effect clinically important (irrespective of whether or not the result of the relevant hypothesis test is statistically significant) if the lower limit of the confidence interval represented the true value of the effect?
  (ii) Would you regard the observed effect clinically important if the upper limit of the confidence interval represented the true value of the effect?
  (iii) Are your answers to the above two points sufficiently similar to declare the results of the study unambiguous and important?

- To assess therapy in a randomized controlled trial, evaluate the **number of patients you need to treat** (NNT) with the experimental treatment rather than the control treatment in order to prevent one of them developing the 'bad' outcome (such as post-partum haemorrhage, see Example). The NNT can be determined in various ways depending on the information available. It is, for example, the reciprocal of the difference in the proportions of individuals with the bad outcome in the control and experimental groups (see Example).

5   Apply the results in clinical practice

If the results are to help you in caring for your patients, you must ensure that:

• your patient is similar to those on whom the results were obtained;
• the results can be applied to your patient;
• all clinically important outcomes have been considered;

• the likely benefits are worth the potential harms and costs.

6   Evaluate your performance

Self-evaluation involves questioning your abilities to complete tasks 1 to 5 successfully. Are you then able to integrate the critical appraisal into clinical practice, and have you audited your performance? You should also ask yourself whether you have learnt from past experience so that you are now more efficient and are finding the whole process of EBM easier.

Example

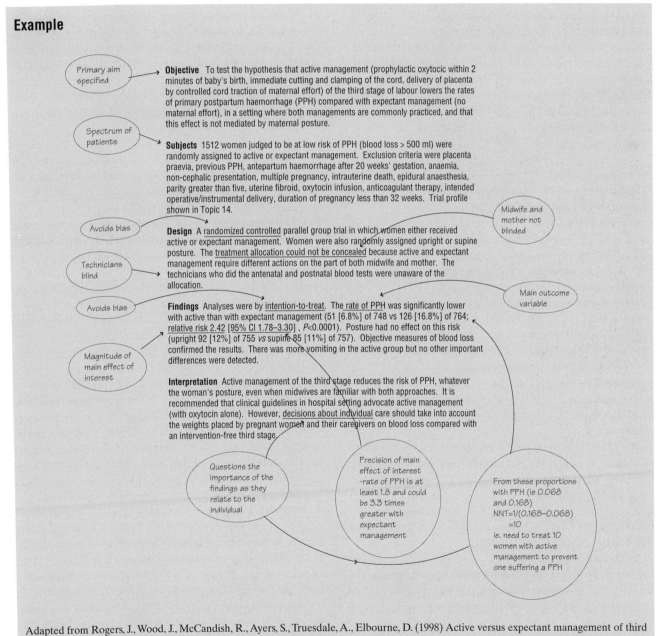

Adapted from Rogers, J., Wood, J., McCandish, R., Ayers, S., Truesdale, A., Elbourne, D. (1998) Active versus expectant management of third stage of labour: the Hinchingbrooke randomised controlled trial. *Lancet*, **351**, 693–699, with permission.

38 Systematic reviews and meta-analysis

The systematic review

What is it?

A **systematic review**[1] is a formalized and stringent process of combining the information from *all* relevant studies (both published and unpublished) of the same health condition; these studies are usually clinical trials (Topic 14) of the same or similar treatments but may be observational studies (Topics 15 and 16). Clearly, a systematic review is an integral part of **evidence based medicine** (EBM; Topic 37), which applies the results of the best available evidence, together with clinical expertise, to the care of patients. So important is its role in EBM, that it has become the focus of an international network of clinicians, methodologists and consumers who have formed the **Cochrane Collaboration**. They have created the Cochrane Controlled Trials Register, and publish continually updated systematic reviews in various forms (e.g. on CD ROM).

What does it achieve?

- **Refinement and reduction**—large quantities of information are refined and reduced to a manageable size.
- **Efficiency**—the systematic review is usually quicker and less costly to perform than a new study. It may prevent others embarking on unnecessary studies, and can shorten the time lag between medical developments and their implementation.
- **Generalizability and consistency**—results can often be generalized to a wider patient population in a broader setting than would be possible from a single study. Consistencies in the results from different studies can be assessed, and any inconsistencies determined.
- **Reliability**—the systematic review aims to reduce errors, and so tends to improve the reliability and accuracy of recommendations when compared with haphazard reviews or single studies.
- **Power and precision**—the quantitative systematic review (see meta-analysis) has greater power (Topic 18) to detect effects of interest and provides more precise estimates of them than a single study.

Meta-analysis

What is it?

A **meta-analysis** or **overview** is a particular type of systematic review that focuses on the numerical results. The main aim of a meta-analysis is to combine the results from individual studies to produce, if appropriate, an estimate of

the overall or average effect of interest (e.g. the relative risk, RR; Topic 15). The direction and magnitude of this average effect, together with a consideration of the associated confidence interval and hypothesis test result, can be used to make decisions about the therapy under investigation and the management of patients.

Statistical approach

1. We decide on the **effect of interest** and, if the raw data are available, evaluate it for each study. However, in practice, we may have to extract these effects from published results. If the outcome in a clinical trial comparing two treatments is:

- **numerical**—the effect may be the difference in treatment means. A zero difference implies no treatment effect;
- **binary** (e.g. died/survived)—we consider the risks of the outcome (e.g. death) in the treatment groups. The effect may be the difference in risks or their ratio, the RR. If the difference in risks equals zero or $RR = 1$ then there is no treatment effect.

2. Obtain an estimate of statistical heterogeneity and check for statistical homogeneity—we have **statistical heterogeneity** when there is considerable variation between the estimates of the effect of interest from the different studies. We can measure it, and perform a hypothesis test to investigate whether the individual estimates are compatible (i.e. homogeneous). If there is significant statistical heterogeneity, we should proceed cautiously, investigate the reasons for its presence and modify our approach accordingly.

3. Estimate the average effect of interest (with a confidence interval), and perform the appropriate hypothesis test on the effect (e.g. that the true $RR = 1$)—you may come across the terms 'fixed-effects' and 'random-effects' models in this context. Although the underlying concepts are beyond the scope of this book, note that we generally use a fixed-effects model if there is no evidence of statistical heterogeneity, and a random-effects model otherwise.

4. Interpret the results and present the findings—it is helpful to summarize the results from each trial (e.g. the sample size, baseline characteristics, effect of interest such as the RR, and related confidence intervals, CI) in a table (see Example). The most common graphical display is a **forest plot** (Fig. 38.1) in which the estimated effect (with CI) for each trial, and their average, are marked along the length of a vertical line which represents 'no treatment effect' (e.g. this line corresponds to the value 'one' if the effect is a RR). Initially, we examine whether the estimated

[1] Chalmers, I. & Altman, D.G. (eds) (1995) *Systematic Reviews.* British Medical Journal Publishing Group, London.

effects from the different studies are on the same side of the line. Then we can use the CIs to judge whether the results are compatible (if the CIs overlap), to determine whether incompatible results can be explained by small sample sizes (if CIs are wide) and to assess the significance of the individual and overall effects (by observing whether the vertical line crosses some or all of the CIs).

Advantages and disadvantages

As a meta-analysis is a particular form of systematic review, it offers all the **advantages** of the latter (see 'what does it achieve?'). In particular, a meta-analysis, because of its inflated sample size, is able to detect treatment effects with **greater power** and estimate these effects with **greater precision** than any single study. Its advantages, together with the introduction of meta-analysis software, have led meta-analyses to proliferate. However, improper use can lead to erroneous conclusions regarding treatment effi-cacy. The following principal **problems** should be thoroughly investigated and resolved before a meta-analysis is performed.

- **Publication bias**—the tendency to include in the analysis only the results from published papers; these favour statistically significant findings.
- **Clinical heterogeneity**—in which differences in the patient population, outcome measures, definition of variables, and/or duration of follow-up of the studies included in the analysis create problems of non-compatibility.
- **Quality differences**—the design and conduct of the studies may vary in their quality. Although giving more weight to the better studies is one solution to this dilemma, any weighting system can be criticized on the grounds that it is arbitrary.
- **Dependence**—the results from studies included in the analysis may not be independent, e.g. when results from a study are published on more than one occasion.

Example

A patient with severe angina will often be eligible for either percutaneous transluminal coronary angioplasty (PTCA) or coronary artery bypass graft (CABG) surgery. Results from eight published randomized trials were combined in a collaborative meta-analysis of 3371 patients (1661 CABG, 1710 PTCA) with a mean follow-up of 2.7 years. The main features of the trials are shown in Table 38.1. Results for the composite endpoint of cardiac death plus non-fatal myocardial infarction (MI) in the first year of follow-up are shown in Fig. 38.1. The estimated relative

Table 38.1 Characteristics of eight randomized trials comparing percutaneous transluminal coronary angioplasty and coronary artery bypass graft.

	Country	Principal investigator	Single- or multi-vessel	Number of patients		Follow-up (years)
				CABG	PTCA	
Coronary Angioplasty Bypass Revascularisation Investigation (CABRI)	Europe	A.F. Rickards	Multi	513	541	1
Randomised Intervention on Treatment of Angina Trial (RITA)	UK	J.R. Hampton	Single ($n = 456$) and multi ($n = 555$)	501	510	4.7
Emory Angioplasty versus Surgery Trial (EAST)	USA	S.B. King	Multi	194	198	3+
German Angioplasty Bypass Surgery Investigation (GABI)	Germany	C.W. Hamm	Multi	177	182	1
The Toulouse Trial (Toulouse)	France	J. Puel	Multi	76	76	2.8
Medicine Angioplasty or Surgery study (MASS)	Brazil	W. Hueb	Single	70	72	3.2
The Lausanne trial (Lausanne)	Switzerland	J.-J. Goy	Single	66	68	3.2
Argentine Trial of PTCA versus CABG (ERACI)	Argentina	A. Rodriguez	Multi	64	63	3.8

continued

risks (RR) are for the PTCA group compared with the CABG group. The figure uses a logarithmic scale for the RR to achieve symmetrical confidence intervals (CI). Although the individual estimates of relative risk vary quite considerably, from reductions in risk to quite large increases in risk, all the confidence intervals overlap to some extent. The RR = 1.03 for all trials combined (95% CI 0.79–1.50), indicating that there was no evidence of an overall difference between the two revascularization strategies. It may be of interest to note that during early follow-up the prevalence of angina was higher in PTCA patients than in CABG patients.

	No. (and %) having cardiac death or MI in first year	
Trial	CABG	PTCA
CABRI	29 (5.7%)	43 (7.9%)
RITA	31 (6.2%)	34 (6.7%)
EAST	33 (18.4%)	24 (13.7%)
GABI	18 (10.2%)	10 (5.5%)
Toulouse	6 (7.9%)	6 (7.9%)
MASS	1 (1.4%)	5 (6.9%)
Lausanne	2 (3.0%)	6 (8.8%)
ERACI	7 (10.9%)	8 (12.7%)
All trials	127	135

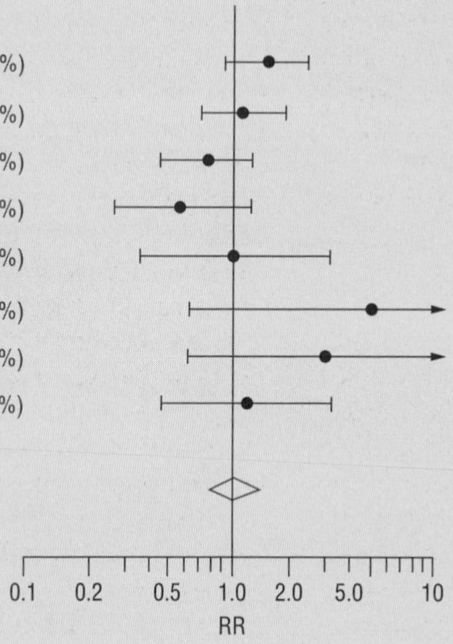

Fig. 38.1 Forest plot of RR (95% CI) of cardiac death or myocardial infarction for PTCA group compared with CABG group in first year since randomization.

Adapted from Pocock, S.J., Henderson, R.A., Rickards A.F., *et al.* (1995) A meta-analysis of randomised trials comparing coronary angioplasty with bypass surgery. *Lancet*, **346**, 1184–1189, with permission.

39 Methods for repeated measures

Often we have a numerical variable that is measured in each member of a group of individuals in different circumstances. We shall assume the circumstances are different time points but they could, for example, be doses of a drug or teeth in a mouth. Such data are known as **repeated measures** data, and are a generalization of paired data (Topic 20). Where the circumstances represent different time points, we have a special type of **longitudinal data**; other types of longitudinal data include time series (Topic 40) and survival data (Topic 41). We summarize repeated measures data by describing the patterns in individuals, and, if relevant, assess whether these patterns differ between two or more groups of individuals.

Displaying the data

A plot of the measurement against time (say) for each individual in the study provides a visual impression of the pattern over time. When we are studying only a small group of patients, it may be possible to show all the individual plots in one diagram. However, when we are studying large groups this becomes difficult, and we may illustrate just a selection of 'representative' individual plots (Fig. 39.1), perhaps in a grid for each treatment group. Note that the average pattern generated by plotting the means over all individuals at each time point may be very different from the patterns seen in individuals.

Inappropriate analyses

It is **inappropriate** to fit a *single* linear regression line (Topics 27, 28) or perform a one-way analysis of variance (ANOVA) (Topic 22) using all values because these methods do not take account of the repeated measurements on the same individual. Furthermore, it is also **incorrect** to compare the means in the groups *at each time point separately* using unpaired *t*-tests (Topic 21) or one-way ANOVA (Topic 22), for a number of reasons:
- The measurements in an individual from one time point to the next are not independent, so interpretation of the results is difficult. For example, if a comparison is significant at one time point, then it is likely to be significant at subsequent time points, irrespective of any changes in the values in the interim period.
- The large number of tests carried out implies that we are likely to obtain significant results purely by chance (Topic 18).
- We lose information about within-patient changes.

Appropriate analyses
Using summary measures

We can base our analysis on a **summary measure** that captures the important aspects of the data, and calculate this summary measure for each individual. Typical summary measures are:
- change from baseline at a pre-determined timepoint;
- maximum (peak) or minimum (nadir) value reached;
- time to reach the maximum (or minimum) value;
- time to reach some other pre-specified value;
- average value;
- area under the curve (AUC, Fig. 39.2).

The choice of summary measure depends on the main question of interest and should be made in advance of collecting the data. For example, if we are considering drug concentrations after treatment with two therapies, we may choose time to maximum drug concentration (C_{max}) or AUC. However, if we are interested in antibody titres after vaccination, then we may choose the time it takes the antibody titre to drop below a particular protective level.

We compare the values of the summary measure in the different groups using standard hypothesis tests [e.g. Wilcoxon rank sum (Topic 21) or Kruskal–Wallis (Topic 22)]. Because we have reduced a number of dependent measurements on each individual to a single quantity, the values included in the analysis are now independent.

Although analyses based on summary measures are simple to perform, it may be difficult to find a suitable measure that adequately describes the data, and we may need to use two or more summary measures. In addition, these approaches do not use all data values fully.

The use of regression parameters as summary measures
It may be possible to find a particular **regression model** (Topics 27–29) that describes the relationship (e.g. linear or quadratic) between the measurement and time. We can estimate the parameters of this model separately *for each individual*. One of the **coefficients** of this model (e.g. the *slope* or *intercept* when modelling the relationship as a straight line) can be used as a summary measure. However, there are sometimes problems with this approach, such as the coefficients being estimated with different levels of precision. For example, the slope for an individual with only three measurements may be estimated much less precisely than that for an individual with 20 measurements. This can lead to misleading results, unless we take account of it in any analysis by putting more weight on those measures that are estimated more precisely.

Repeated measures analysis of variance

We can perform a particular type of ANOVA (Topic 22), called **repeated measures ANOVA**, in which the different time points are considered as the levels of one factor in the analysis and the grouping variable is a second factor in the analysis. If this analysis produces significant differences between the groups, then adjusted t-tests, which take account of the dependence in the data, can be performed to identify at what time points these differences become apparent[1].

However, repeated measures ANOVA has several disadvantages.
- It is often difficult to perform.
- The results may be difficult to interpret.
- It generally assumes that values are measured at regular time intervals and that there are no missing data, i.e. the

design of the study is assumed to be **balanced**. In reality, values are rarely measured at all time points because patients often miss appointments or come at different times to those planned.

Multi-level modelling

Multi-level modelling[2], a hierarchical extension of regression, also provides a means of analysing repeated measures data. There is no requirement for the design to be balanced, and individuals for whom very few measurements are available benefit from 'shared' information, because their estimates are based not only on their own values, but also on the patterns that are seen in the other individuals in the study. Therefore, these methods provide a powerful way of testing for differences between groups, but they are complex and require specialist computer software.

[1] Hand, D.J. & Taylor, C.C. (1987) *Multivariate Analysis of Variance and Repeated Measures.* Chapman and Hall, London.

[2] Goldstein, H. (1987) *Multilevel Models in Educational and Social Research.* Charles Griffin and Company Ltd., London.

Example

As part of a practical class designed to assess the effects of two inhaled bronchodilator drugs, fenoterol hydrobromide and ipratropium bromide, 99 medical students were randomized to receive one of these drugs ($n = 33$ for each drug) or placebo ($n = 33$). Each student inhaled four times in quick succession. Tremor was assessed by measuring the total time (in seconds) taken to thread five sewing needles mounted on a cork; measurements were made at baseline before inhalation and at 5, 15, 30, 45 and 60 mins afterwards. The measurements of a representative sample of the students in each treatment group are shown in Fig. 39.1.

It was decided to compare the values in the three groups using the 'area under the curve' (AUC) as a summary measure. The calculation of AUC for one student is illustrated in Fig. 39.2.

The median (range) AUC were 1552.5 (417.5–3875), 1215 (457.5–2500) and 1130 (547.5–2625) seconds[2] in those receiving fenoterol hydrobromide, ipratropium bromide and placebo, respectively. The values in the three groups were compared using the Kruskal–Wallis test which gave $P = 0.008$. There was thus strong evidence that the AUC measures were different in the three groups. Non-parametric *post-hoc* comparisons indicated that values were greater in the group receiving fenoterol hydrobromide, confirming pharmacological knowledge that this drug, as a β_2-adrenoceptor agonist, induces tremor by the stimulation of β_2-adrenoceptors in skeletal muscle.

Data were kindly provided by Dr R. Morris, Department of Primary Care and Population Sciences, and were collected as part of a student practical class organized by Dr T.J. Allen, Department of Pharmacology, Royal Free and University College Medical School, Royal Free Campus, London; UK.

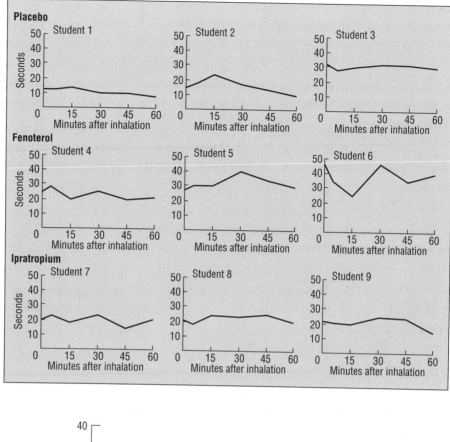

Fig. 39.1 Time taken to thread five sewing needles for three representative students in each treatment group.

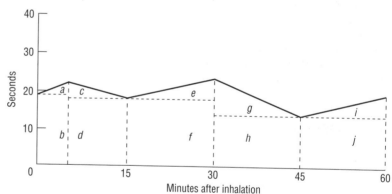

Fig. 39.2 Calculation of the AUC for a single student. The total area under the line can be divided into a number of rectangles and triangles (marked a to j). The area of each can easily be calculated. Total AUC = Area (a) + Area (b) + ... + Area (j).

40 Time series

A **time series** consists of a series of single values (e.g. incidence) at each of many time points (Fig. 40.1), and is a particular type of longitudinal data. For example, we may have monthly incidence rates of an infectious disease. The time period over which the values are available is reasonably long relative to the frequency of measurement, enabling trends and seasonal patterns to be discerned. It is distinguished from repeated measures data (Topic 39), which usually shows *all* the measurements taken on *each* of a number of individuals at perhaps only a few time points. A time series may be **discrete** with measurements taken at specified time intervals (e.g. hourly or yearly), or may be **continuous**, such as that obtained from machines that continuously monitor patients' vital signs.

Components of a time series
Time series often show one or more of the following features.
- **Trend**—values have a tendency to increase or decrease over time (Fig. 40.2). For example, the annual number of reported episodes of food poisoning has increased over time.
- **Seasonal variation**—similar patterns appear in corresponding seasons in successive years (Fig. 40.2). For example, hay fever rates show a distinct seasonal pattern.
- **Other cyclic variation**—variation of any other fixed period. For example, measurements may display a circadean pattern, with levels cycling over a 24 h period.
- **Random variation**—variation that does not exhibit any fixed pattern over time (Fig. 40.2).
- **Serial correlation**—observations close together in the time series are highly correlated, even after adjusting for any trend and/or cyclic variation. For example, a high

number of reported 'flu cases on any day is likely to be followed by high numbers of reported cases on subsequent days.

A plot of the values against time will usually identify whether the time series exhibits any of these components, as well as highlighting any outliers.

Analysing time series data
We usually have one of two **aims** when studying time series data.
- To understand the mechanism that generated the series in order to produce a model that can be used to *predict* future values of the series.
- To assess the impact of some *exposure* on the series, after taking account of confounding variables. For example, we may wish to assess the impact of air pollution, measurements which themselves form a time series, on the number of asthma attacks, after taking account of daily weather conditions. If we are concerned with the relationship between two series which show a similar trend (e.g. a seasonal trend, or a gradual increase over time), then the two series will be correlated, even if there is no underlying causal relationship between them. Therefore, we must remove any trend and/or cyclic variation before assessing the relationship or the role of an exposure.

For the purposes of analysis, we usually reduce our time series to a **stationary time series**, in which there is no trend and cyclic variation does not increase or decrease over time.

Generating the model
We start by creating a model that explicitly incorporates any trend (by including 'time' and/or 'time^2' as a factor in

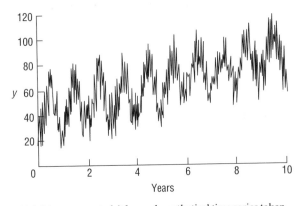

Fig. 40.1 Measurements (y) from a hypothetical time series taken over a period of 10 years.

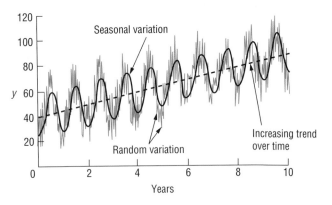

Fig. 40.2 The effects of trend, seasonal variation and random variation on the time series shown in Fig. 40.1.

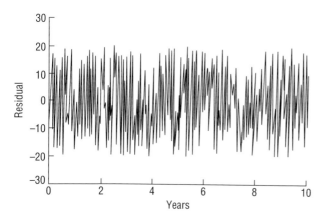

Fig. 40.3 Random component of time series after removing trend and seasonal variation.

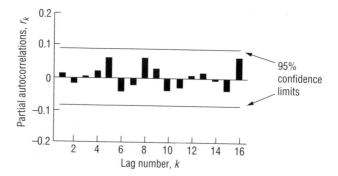

Fig. 40.4 Partial autocorrelation function of the time series of residual values obtained after removing trend and seasonality. None of the partial autocorrelations lies outside the 95% confidence limits, indicating that no large autocorrelation remains in the residual series.

the model). Sometimes we may also need to take a transformation (e.g. logs, Topic 9) to satisfy the assumptions underlying the model (e.g. constant variance). The residuals from this model (i.e. the observed value minus the value predicted from the model at each time point) themselves form a time series that will be stationary.

We then identify the presence and frequency of any cyclic variation in this residual series (see next section); this is incorporated into the model, usually by including sine and cosine terms, as appropriate.

Because of the serial correlation in the series, measurements at successive time points are not independent. Therefore, we use special regression methods[1] (e.g. **autoregressive** models) that allow for the dependence of the values.

We assess whether the model is a good description of the time series by considering the residuals of the model. If the current model is satisfactory, the residuals will be a **random series** with no discernible trends or cyclic variation (Fig. 40.3). If we do not have a random series of residuals, then we include other factors, if possible, in the model and repeat the process.

If our aim is prediction, then we use the time series model to predict values at future time points. If, however, we want to assess the impact of some exposure on the time series, we use the time series of the residuals in any subsequent analysis. We then use modelling processes specific to time series data, for example, **moving average** models, to assess the impact of the exposure.

Identifying cyclic variation

Cyclic variation in the data can often be judged visually, although this may be difficult to assess if there is substantial random fluctuation in the series. Two complementary approaches, based on the correlogram or periodogram, can be used to identify cyclic patterns in the residual time series obtained after modelling the trend and/or taking transformations.

The correlogram

This is especially useful for assessing cyclic variation of *short periods*, and focuses on the relationships between observations different time periods apart (**serial correlation**). This relationship is described by the **autocorrelation coefficient** of lag k (referred to as r_k), which measures the correlation between observations k time units apart. A plot of r_k against values of k, known as the **correlogram**, illustrates the **autocorrelation** structure of the data. If there is no autocorrelation (i.e. r_k is approximately equal to zero for all non-zero values of k), then we have a random series. High autocorrelation at certain lags (e.g. $k = 12$ or 24 when measuring hourly data) may indicate the presence of cyclic variation. More usually, we consider the **partial autocorrelation function**, by plotting the autocorrelation at each lag, after correcting for autocorrelation at earlier lags, against k (Fig. 40.4). A high partial autocorrelation coefficient at a particular value of k suggests the possibility of cyclic variation at that lag, which can then be incorporated into the model.

The periodogram

This is especially useful for assessing cyclic variation of longer frequencies. A special graphical display of the residual series, known as the **periodogram**, is used to identify the frequency and period of cycles in the original series.

[1] Chatfield, C. (1984) *The Analysis of Time Series*. Chapman and Hall, London.

41 Survival analysis

Survival data are concerned with the time it takes an individual to reach an endpoint of interest (often, but not always, death) and are characterized by the following two features.
- It is the **length of time** for the patient to reach the endpoint, rather than whether or not he/she reaches the endpoint, that is of primary importance. For example, we may be interested in length of survival in patients admitted with cirrhosis.
- Data may often be **censored** (see below).

Standard methods of analysis, such as logistic regression or a comparison of the mean time to reaching the endpoint in patients with and without a new treatment, can give misleading results because of the censored data. Therefore, a number of statistical techniques, known as **survival methods**[1], have been developed to deal with these situations.

Censored data

Survival times are calculated from some baseline date that reflects a natural 'starting point' for the study (e.g. time of surgery or diagnosis of a condition) until the time that a patient reaches the endpoint of interest. Often, however, we may not know when the patient reached the endpoint, only that he/she remained free of the endpoint while in the study. For example, patients in a trial of a new drug for HIV infection may remain AIDS-free when they leave the study. This may either be because the trial ended while they were still AIDS-free, or because these individuals withdrew from the trial early before developing AIDS, or because they died of non-AIDS causes before the end of follow-up. Such data are described as **right-censored**. These patients were known *not* to have reached the endpoint when they were last under follow-up, and this information should be incorporated into the analysis.

Where follow-up does not begin until after the baseline date, survival times can also be **left-censored**.

Displaying survival data

- A separate horizontal line can be drawn for each patient, its length indicating the survival time. Lines are drawn from left to right, and patients who reach the endpoint and those who are censored can be distinguished by the use of different symbols at the end of the line (Fig. 41.1). However, these plots do not summarize the data and it is difficult to get a feel for the survival experience overall.
- **Survival curves**, usually calculated by the **Kaplan–Meier** method, display the cumulative probability (the **survival probability**) of an individual remaining free of the endpoint at any time after baseline (Fig. 41.2). The survival probability will only change when an endpoint occurs, and thus the resulting 'curve' is drawn as a series of steps. An alternative method of calculating survival probabilities, using a **lifetable** approach, can be used when the time to reach the endpoint is only known to within a particular time interval (e.g. within a year). The survival probabilities using either method are simple but time-consuming to calculate, and can be easily obtained from most statistical packages.

Summarizing survival

We often summarize survival by quoting survival probabilities (with confidence intervals) at certain time points on the curve, for example, the 5 year survival rates in patients after treatment for breast cancer. Alternatively, the median time to reach the endpoint (the time at which 50% of the individuals have *progressed*) can be quoted.

Comparing survival

We may wish to assess the impact of a number of factors of interest on survival, e.g. treatment, disease severity. Survival curves can be plotted separately for subgroups of patients; they provide a means of assessing visually whether different groups of patients reach the endpoint at different rates (Fig. 41.2). We can test formally whether there are any significant differences in progression rates between the different groups by, for example, using the log-rank test or regression models.

The log-rank test

This non-parametric test addresses the null hypothesis that there are no differences in survival times in the groups being studied, and compares events occurring at all time points on the survival curve. We cannot assess the independent roles of more than one factor on the time to the endpoint using the log-rank test.

Regression models

We can generate a regression model to quantify the relationships between one or more factors of interest and survival. At any point in time, t, an individual, i, has an instantaneous risk of reaching the endpoint (often known as the **hazard**, or $\lambda_i(t)$), given that he/she has not reached it up to that point in time. For example, if death is the endpoint, the hazard is the risk of dying at time t. This instantaneous hazard is usually very small and is of limited interest. However, we may want to know whether there are any systematic differences between the hazards, over all time

[1] Cox, D.R., Oakes, D. (1984) *Analysis of Survival Data*. Chapman and Hall, London.

points, of individuals with different characteristics. For example, is the hazard generally reduced in individuals treated with a new therapy compared with those treated with a placebo, when we take into account other factors, such as age or disease severity?

• We can use the **Cox proportional hazards model** to test the independent effects of a number of explanatory variables (factors) on the hazard. It is of the form:

$$\lambda_i(t) = \lambda_0(t)\exp\{\beta_1 x_1 + \beta_2 x_2 + \ldots + \beta_n x_n\}$$

where $\lambda_i(t)$ is the hazard for individual i at time t, $\lambda_0(t)$ is an arbitrary baseline hazard (in which we are not interested), $x_1 \ldots x_n$ are explanatory variables in the model and $\beta_1 \ldots \beta_n$ are the corresponding coefficients. We obtain estimates, $b_1 \ldots b_n$, of these parameters using specialized computer programs. The exponential of these values (e^{b_1}, e^{b_2}, etc.) are known as the estimated **relative hazards** or **hazard ratios**; each represents the increased or decreased risk of reaching the endpoint at any point in time associated with a unit increase in its associated x (i.e. x_1, or x_2, etc.), adjusting for the other explanatory variables in the model. The relative hazard is interpreted in a similar manner to the odds ratio in logistic regression (Topic 30); therefore values above one indicate a raised risk, values below one indicate a decreased risk and values equal to one indicate that there is no increased or decreased risk of the endpoint. A confidence interval can be calculated for the relative hazard and a significance test performed to assess its departure from 1.

The relative hazard is assumed to be constant over time in this model (i.e. the hazards for the groups to be compared are assumed to be *proportional*). It is important to check this assumption either by using graphical methods or by incorporating an interaction between the covariate and log(time) in the model and ensuring that it is non-significant[1].

• Other models can be used to describe survival data, e.g. the **Exponential** or **Weibull** model. However, these are beyond the scope of this book[1].

Example

Height of portal pressure (HVPG) is known to be associated with the severity of alcoholic cirrhosis but is rarely used as a predictor of survival in patients with cirrhosis. In order to assess the clinical value of this measurement, 105 patients admitted to hospital with cirrhosis, undergoing hepatic venography, were followed for a median of 566 days. The experience of these patients is illustrated in Fig. 41.1. Over the follow-up period, 33 patients died. Kaplan–Meier curves showing the cumulative survival rate at any time point after baseline are displayed separately for individuals in whom HVPG was less than 16 mmHg (a value previously suggested to provide prognostic significance) and for those in whom HVPG was 16 mmHg or greater (Fig. 41.2).

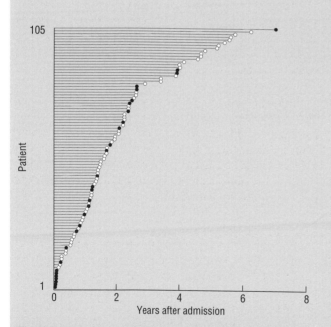

Fig. 41.1 Survival experience in 105 patients following admission with cirrhosis. Filled circles indicate patients who died, open circles indicate those who remained alive at the end of follow-up.

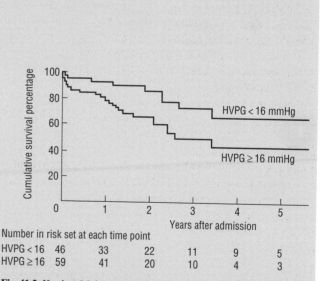

Number in risk set at each time point

HVPG < 16	46	33	22	11	9	5
HVPG ≥ 16	59	41	20	10	4	3

Fig. 41.2 Kaplan–Meier curves showing the survival probability, expressed as a percentage, following admission for cirrhosis, stratified by baseline HVPG measurement.

continued

The computer output for the log-rank test contained the following information:

Test	Chi-square	df	P-value
Log-rank	5.2995	1	0.0213

Thus there is a significant difference ($P = 0.02$) between survival times in the two groups. By 3 years after admission, 73.1% of those with a low HVPG measurement remained alive, compared with 49.6% of those with a higher measurement (Fig. 41.2).

A Cox proportional hazards regression model was used to investigate whether this relationship could be explained by differences in any known prognostic or demographic factors at baseline. Twenty variables were considered for inclusion in the model, including demographic, clinical and laboratory markers. Graphical methods suggested that the proportional hazards assumption was reasonable for these variables. A stepwise selection procedure (Topic 31) was used to select the final optimal model, and the results are shown in Table 41.1.

The results in Table 41.1 indicate that raised HVPG remains independently associated with shorter survival after adjusting for other factors known to be associated with a poorer outcome. In particular, individuals with HVPG of 16 mmHg or higher had 2.46 ($=\exp\{0.90\}$) times the hazard of death compared with those with lower levels ($P = 0.04$) after adjusting for other factors. In other words, the hazard of death is increased by 146% in these individuals. In addition, increased prothrombin time (hazard increases by 5% per additional second), increased bilirubin level (hazard increases by 5% per 10 additional mmol/L), the presence of ascites (hazard increases by 126% for increase in level) and previous long-term endoscopic treatment (hazard increases by 246%) were all independently associated with outcome.

Table 41.1 Results of Cox proportional hazards regression model.

Variable (and coding)	df	Parameter estimate	Standard error	P-value	Relative hazard	95% CI for relative hazard
HVPG* (0 = <16, 1 = ≥16 mmHg)	1	0.90	0.44	0.04	2.46	(1.03–5.85)
Prothrombin time (secs)	1	0.05	0.01	0.0002	1.05	(1.02–1.07)
Bilirubin (10 mmol/L)	1	0.05	0.02	0.04	1.05	(1.00–1.10)
Ascites (0 = none, 1 = mild, 2 = moderate/severe)	1	0.82	0.18	0.0001	2.26	(1.58–3.24)
Previous long-term endoscopic treatment (0 = no, 1 = yes)	1	1.24	0.41	0.003	3.46	(1.54–7.76)

HVPG*, Height of portal pressure.

Data kindly provided by Dr D. Patch and Dr A.K. Burroughs, Liver Unit, Royal Free Hospital, London, UK.

42 Bayesian methods

The frequentist approach

The hypothesis tests described in this book are based on the **frequentist** approach to probability (Topic 7) and inference that considers the number of times an event would occur if we were to repeat the experiment a large number of times. This approach is sometimes criticized for the following reasons.

- It uses only information obtained from the current study, and does not incorporate into the inferential process any other information we might have about the effect of interest, e.g. a clinician's views about the relative effectiveness of two therapies before a clinical trial is undertaken.
- It does not directly address the issues of greatest interest. In a drug comparison, we are really interested in knowing whether one drug is *more effective* than the other. However, the frequentist approach tests the hypothesis that the two drugs are *equally effective*. Although we conclude that one drug is superior to the other if the *P*-value is small, this probability (i.e. the *P*-value) describes the chance of getting the observed results if the drugs are equally effective, rather than the chance that one drug is more effective than the other (our real interest).
- It tends to over-emphasize the role of hypothesis testing and whether or not a result is significant, rather than the implications of the results.

The Bayesian approach

An alternative, **Bayesian**[1], approach to inference reflects an individual's personal degree of belief in a hypothesis, possibly based on information already available. Individuals usually differ in their degrees of belief in a hypothesis; in addition, these beliefs may change as new information becomes available. The Bayesian approach calculates the probability that a hypothesis is *true* (our focus of interest) by updating *prior* opinions about the hypothesis as new data become available.

Conditional probability

A particular type of probability, known as **conditional probability**, is fundamental to Bayesian analyses. This is the probability of an event, given that another event has already occurred. As an illustration, consider an example. The incidence of haemophilia A in the general population is approximately 1 in 10 000 male births. However, if we know that a woman is a carrier for haemophilia, this incidence increases to around 1 in 2 male births. Therefore, the probability that a male child has haemophilia, given that his mother is a carrier, is very different to the unconditional probability that he has haemophilia if his mother's carrier status is unknown.

Bayes theorem

Suppose we are investigating a hypothesis (e.g. that a treatment effect equals some value). Bayes theorem converts a **prior probability**, describing an individual's belief in the hypothesis *before* the study is carried out, into a **posterior probability**, describing his/her beliefs *afterwards*. The posterior probability is, in fact, the conditional probability of the hypothesis, given the results from the study. **Bayes theorem** states that the **posterior probability** is proportional to the **prior probability** multiplied by a value, the **likelihood** of the observed results, which describes the plausibility of the observed results if the hypothesis is true.

Diagnostic tests in a Bayesian framework

Almost all clinicians intuitively use a Bayesian approach in their reasoning when making a diagnosis. They build a picture of the patient based on clinical history and/or the presence of symptoms and signs. From this, they decide on the *most likely* diagnosis, having eliminated other diagnoses on the presumption that they are unlikely to be true, given what they know about the patient. They may subsequently confirm or amend this diagnosis in the light of new evidence, e.g. if the patient responds to treatment or a new symptom develops.

When an individual attends a clinic, the clinician usually has some idea of the probability that the individual has the disease—the **prior** or **pre-test probability**. If nothing else is known about the patient, this is simply the **prevalence** (Topics 12 and 35) of the disease in the population. We can use Bayes theorem to change the prior probability into a posterior probability. This is most easily achieved if we incorporate the **likelihood ratio**, based on information obtained from the most recent investigation (e.g. a diagnostic test result), into Bayes theorem. The likelihood ratio of a positive test result is the chance of a positive test result if the patient has disease, divided by that if he/she is disease-free. We introduced the likelihood ratio in Topic 35, and showed that it could be used to indicate the usefulness of a diagnostic test. In the same context, we now use it to express Bayes theorem in terms of odds (Topic 16):

Posterior odds of disease = prior odds × likelihood ratio of a positive test result

where

[1] Freedman, L. (1996) Bayesian statistical methods. A natural way to assess clinical evidence. *British Medical Journal*, **313**, 569–570.

$$\text{Prior odds} = \frac{\text{prior probability}}{(1 - \text{prior probability})}$$

$$\text{and likelihood ratio} = \frac{\text{sensitivity}}{1 - \text{specificity}}$$

The posterior odds is simple to calculate, but for easier interpretation, we convert the odds back into a probability using the relationship:

$$\text{Posterior probability} = \frac{\text{posterior odds}}{(1 + \text{posterior odds})}$$

This **posterior** or **post-test probability** is the probability that the patient has the disease, given a positive test result. It is similar to the positive predictive value (Topic 35) but takes account of the prior probability that the individual has the disease.

A simpler way to perform these calculations is to use **Fagan's nomogram** (see Fig. 42.1); by connecting the pre-test probability (expressed as a percentage) to the likelihood ratio and extending the line, we can evaluate the post-test probability.

Disadvantages of Bayesian methods

As part of any Bayesian analysis, it is necessary to specify the prior probability of the hypothesis (e.g. the pre-test probability that a patient has disease). Because of the subjective nature of these priors, individual researchers and clinicians may choose different values for them. For this reason, Bayesian methods are often criticized as being arbitrary. Where the most recent evidence from the study (i.e. the likelihood) is very strong, however, the influence of the prior information is minimized (at its extreme, the results will be completely uninfluenced by the prior information).

The calculations involved in many Bayesian analyses are complex, usually requiring sophisticated statistical packages that are highly computer intensive. Therefore, despite being intuitively appealing, Bayesian methods have not been used widely. However, the availability of powerful

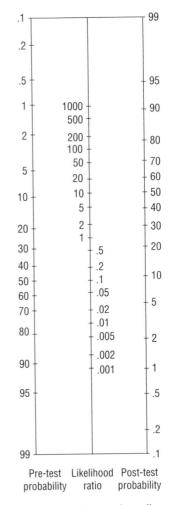

Fig. 42.1 Fagan's nomogram for interpreting a diagnostic test result. Adapted from Sackett, D.L., Richardson, W.S., Rosenberg, W., Haynes, R.B. (1997) *Evidence-based Medicine: How to Practice and Teach EBM*. Churchill-Livingstone, London, with permission.

personal computers means that their use is becoming more common.

Example

In the example in Topic 35 we showed that in bone marrow transplant recipients, a viral load above $5 \log_{10}$ genomes/mL gave the optimal sensitivity and specificity of a test to predict the development of severe clinical disease. The likelihood ratio for a positive test for this cut-off value was 13.3.

If we believe that the prevalence of severe disease as a result of cytomegalovirus (CMV) infection after bone marrow transplantation is approximately 33%, the prior probability of severe disease in these patients equals 0.33.

$$\text{Prior odds} = \frac{0.33}{0.67} = 0.493$$

$$\begin{aligned}\text{Posterior odds} &= 0.493 \times \text{likelihood ratio} \\ &= 0.493 \times 13.3 \\ &= 6.557\end{aligned}$$

$$\text{Posterior probability} = \frac{6.557}{(1+6.557)} = \frac{6.557}{7.557} = 0.868$$

Therefore, if the individual has a CMV viral load above

continued

5 $\log_{10}$ genomes/mL, and we assume that the pre-test probability of severe disease is 0.33, then we believe that the individual has an 87% chance of developing severe disease. This can also be estimated directly from Fagan's nomogram (Fig. 42.1) by connecting the pre-test probability of 33% to a likelihood ratio of 13.3 and extending the line to cut the post-test probability axis. In contrast, if we believe that the probability that an individual will get severe disease is only 20% (i.e. pre-test probability equals 0.2), then the post-test probability will equal 77%.

In both cases, the post-test probability is much higher than the pre-test probability, indicating the usefulness of a positive test result. Furthermore, both results indicate that the patient is at high risk of developing severe disease after transplantation and that it may be sensible to start anti-CMV therapy. Therefore, despite having very different prior probabilities, the general conclusion remains the same in each case.

Appendix A: Statistical tables

This appendix contains statistical tables discussed in the text. We have provided only limited *P*-values because data are usually analysed using a computer, and *P*-values are included in its output. Other texts, such as that by Fisher and Yates[1], contain more comprehensive tables. You can also obtain *P*-values directly from some computer packages, given a value of the test statistic. Empty cells in a table are an indication that values do not exist.

Table A1 contains the probability in the two tails of the distribution of a variable, z, which follows the Standard Normal distribution. The *P*-values in Table A1 relate to the absolute values of z, so if z is negative, we ignore its sign. For example, if a test statistic that follows the Standard Normal distribution has the value 1.1, $P = 0.271$.

Table A2 and **Table A3** contain the probability in the two tails of a distribution of a variable that follows the *t*-distribution (Table A2) or the Chi-squared distribution (Table A3) with given degrees of freedom (df). To use Table A2 or Table A3, if the absolute value of the test statistic (with given df) lies between the tabulated values in two columns, then the two-tailed *P*-value lies between the *P*-values specified at the top of these columns. If the test statistic is to the right of the final column, $P < 0.001$; if it is to the left of the second column, $P > 0.10$. For example, (i) Table A2: if the test statistic is 2.62 with $df = 17$, then $0.01 < P < 0.05$; (ii) Table A3: if the test statistic is 2.62 with $df = 17$, then $P < 0.001$.

Table A4 contains often used *P*-values and their corresponding values for z, a variable with a Standard Normal distribution. This table may be used to obtain multipliers for the calculation of confidence intervals (CI) for Normally distributed variables. For example, for a 95% confidence interval, the multiplier is 1.96.

Table A5 contains *P*-values for a variable that follows the *F*-distribution with specified degrees of freedom in the numerator and denominator. When comparing variances (Topic 32), we usually use a two-tailed *P*-value. For the analysis of variance (Topic 22), we use a one-tailed *P*-value. For given degrees of freedom in the numerator and denominator, the test is significant at the level of *P* quoted in the table if the test statistic is greater than the tabulated value. For example, if the test statistic is 2.99 with $df = 5$ in the numerator and $df = 15$ in the denominator, then $P < 0.05$ for a one-tailed test.

Table A6 contains two-tailed *P*-values of the sign test of k responses of a particular type out of a total of n' responses. For a one-sample test, k equals the number of values above (or below) the median (Topic 19). For a paired test, k equals the number of positive (or negative) differences (Topic 20) or the number of preferences for a particular treatment (Topic 23). n' equals the number of values not equal to the median, non-zero differences or actual preferences, as relevant. For example, if we observed three positive differences out of eight non-zero differences, then $P = 0.726$.

Table A7 contains the ranks of the values which determine the upper and lower limits of the approximate 90%, 95% and 99% confidence intervals (CI) for the median. For example, if the sample size is 23, then the limits of the 95% confidence interval are defined by the 7th and 17th ordered values.

For sample sizes greater than 50, find the observations that correspond to the ranks (to the nearest integer) equal to: (i) $n/2 - z\sqrt{n}/2$; and (ii) $1 + n/2 + z\sqrt{n}/2$; where n is the sample size and $z = 1.64$ for a 90% CI, $z = 1.96$ for a 95% CI, and $z = 2.58$ for a 99% CI (the values of z being obtained from the Standard Normal distribution, Table A4). These observations define (i) the lower, and (ii) the upper confidence limits for the median.

Table A8 contains the range of values for the sum of the ranks (T_+ or T_-), which determines significance in the Wilcoxon signed ranks test (Topic 20). If the sum of the ranks of the positive (T_+) or negative (T_-) differences, out of n' non-zero differences, is equal to or outside the tabulated limits, the test is significant at the *P*-value quoted. For example, if there are 16 non-zero differences and $T_+ = 21$, then $0.01 < P < 0.05$.

Table A9 contains the range of values for the sum of the ranks (T), which determines significance for the Wilcoxon rank sum test (Topic 21) at (a) the 5% level and (b) the 1% level. Suppose we have two samples of sizes n_S and n_L, where $n_S \le n_L$. If the sum of the ranks of the group with the smaller sample size, n_S, is equal to or outside the tabulated limits, the test is significant at (a) the 5% level or (b) the 1% level. For example, if $n_S = 6$ and $n_L = 8$, and the sum of the ranks in the group of six observations equals 39, then $P > 0.05$.

[1] Fisher, R.A. & Yates, F. (1963) *Statistical Tables for Biological, Agricultural and Medical Research*, 6th edn. Oliver and Boyd, Edinburgh.

Tables **A10** and **Table A11** contain two-tailed P-values for Pearson's (Table A10) and Spearman's (Table A11) correlation coefficients when testing the null hypothesis that the relevant correlation coefficient is zero (Topic 26). Significance is achieved, for a given sample size, at the stated P-value if the absolute value (i.e. ignoring its sign) of the sample value of the correlation coefficient exceeds the tabulated value. For example, if the sample size equals 24 and Pearson's $r = 0.58$, then $0.001 < P < 0.01$. If the sample size equals 7 and Spearman's $r_s = -0.63$, then $P > 0.05$.

Table A12 contains the digits 0–9 arranged in random order.

Table A1 Standard Normal distribution.

z	2-tailed P-value
0.0	1.000
0.1	0.920
0.2	0.841
0.3	0.764
0.4	0.689
0.5	0.617
0.6	0.549
0.7	0.484
0.8	0.424
0.9	0.368
1.0	0.317
1.1	0.271
1.2	0.230
1.3	0.194
1.4	0.162
1.5	0.134
1.6	0.110
1.7	0.089
1.8	0.072
1.9	0.057
2.0	0.046
2.1	0.036
2.2	0.028
2.3	0.021
2.4	0.016
2.5	0.012
2.6	0.009
2.7	0.007
2.8	0.005
2.9	0.004
3.0	0.003
3.1	0.002
3.2	0.001
3.3	0.001
3.4	0.001
3.5	0.000

Derived using Microsoft Excel Version 5.0.

Table A2 t-distribution.

df	Two-tailed P-value			
	0.10	0.05	0.01	0.001
1	6.314	12.706	63.656	636.58
2	2.920	4.303	9.925	31.600
3	2.353	3.182	5.841	12.924
4	2.132	2.776	4.604	8.610
5	2.015	2.571	4.032	6.869
6	1.943	2.447	3.707	5.959
7	1.895	2.365	3.499	5.408
8	1.860	2.306	3.355	5.041
9	1.833	2.262	3.250	4.781
10	1.812	2.228	3.169	4.587
11	1.796	2.201	3.106	4.437
12	1.782	2.179	3.055	4.318
13	1.771	2.160	3.012	4.221
14	1.761	2.145	2.977	4.140
15	1.753	2.131	2.947	4.073
16	1.746	2.120	2.921	4.015
17	1.740	2.110	2.898	3.965
18	1.734	2.101	2.878	3.922
19	1.729	2.093	2.861	3.883
20	1.725	2.086	2.845	3.850
21	1.721	2.080	2.831	3.819
22	1.717	2.074	2.819	3.792
23	1.714	2.069	2.807	3.768
24	1.711	2.064	2.797	3.745
25	1.708	2.060	2.787	3.725
26	1.706	2.056	2.779	3.707
27	1.703	2.052	2.771	3.689
28	1.701	2.048	2.763	3.674
29	1.699	2.045	2.756	3.660
30	1.697	2.042	2.750	3.646
40	1.684	2.021	2.704	3.551
50	1.676	2.009	2.678	3.496
100	1.660	1.984	2.626	3.390
200	1.653	1.972	2.601	3.340
5000	1.645	1.960	2.577	3.293

Derived using Microsoft Excel Version 5.0.

Table A3 Chi-squared distribution.

df	Two-tailed P-value			
	0.10	0.05	0.01	0.001
1	2.706	3.841	6.635	10.827
2	4.605	5.991	9.210	13.815
3	6.251	7.815	11.345	16.266
4	7.779	9.488	13.277	18.466
5	9.236	11.070	15.086	20.515
6	10.645	12.592	16.812	22.457
7	12.017	14.067	18.475	24.321
8	13.362	15.507	20.090	26.124
9	14.684	16.919	21.666	27.877
10	15.987	18.307	23.209	29.588
11	17.275	19.675	24.725	31.264
12	18.549	21.026	26.217	32.909
13	19.812	22.362	27.688	34.527
14	21.064	23.685	29.141	36.124
15	22.307	24.996	30.578	37.698
16	23.542	26.296	32.000	39.252
17	24.769	27.587	33.409	40.791
18	25.989	28.869	34.805	42.312
19	27.204	30.144	36.191	43.819
20	28.412	31.410	37.566	45.314
21	29.615	32.671	38.932	46.796
22	30.813	33.924	40.289	48.268
23	32.007	35.172	41.638	49.728
24	33.196	36.415	42.980	51.179
25	34.382	37.652	44.314	52.619
26	35.563	38.885	45.642	54.051
27	36.741	40.113	46.963	55.475
28	37.916	41.337	48.278	56.892
29	39.087	42.557	49.588	58.301
30	40.256	43.773	50.892	59.702
40	51.805	55.758	63.691	73.403
50	63.167	67.505	76.154	86.660
60	74.397	79.082	88.379	99.608
70	85.527	90.531	100.43	112.32
80	96.578	101.88	112.33	124.84
90	107.57	113.15	124.12	137.21
100	118.50	124.34	135.81	149.45

Derived using Microsoft Excel Version 5.0.

Table A4 Standard Normal distribution.

	Two-tailed P-value				
	0.50	0.10	0.05	0.01	0.001
Relevant CI	50%	90%	95%	99%	99.9%
z (i.e. CI multiplier)	0.67	1.64	1.96	2.58	3.29

Derived using Microsoft Excel Version 5.0.

Table A6 Sign test.

	k = number of 'positive differences' (see explanation)					
n'	0	1	2	3	4	5
4	0.125	0.624	1.000			
5	0.062	0.376	1.000			
6	0.032	0.218	0.688	1.000		
7	0.016	0.124	0.454	1.000		
8	0.008	0.070	0.290	0.726	1.000	
9	0.004	0.040	0.180	0.508	1.000	
10	0.001	0.022	0.110	0.344	0.754	1.000

Derived using Microsoft Excel Version 5.0.

Table A5 The F-distribution.

df of denominator	2-tailed P-value	1-tailed P-value	Degrees of freedom (df) of the numerator												
			1	2	3	4	5	6	7	8	9	10	15	25	500
1	0.05	0.025	647.8	799.5	864.2	899.6	921.8	937.1	948.2	956.6	963.3	968.6	984.9	998.1	1017.0
1	0.10	0.05	161.4	199.5	215.7	224.6	230.2	234.0	236.8	238.9	240.5	241.9	245.9	249.3	254.1
2	0.05	0.025	38.51	39.00	39.17	39.25	39.30	39.33	39.36	39.37	39.39	39.40	39.43	39.46	39.50
2	0.10	0.05	18.51	19.00	19.16	19.25	19.30	19.33	19.35	19.37	19.38	19.40	19.43	19.46	19.49
3	0.05	0.025	17.44	16.04	15.44	15.10	14.88	14.73	14.62	14.54	14.47	14.42	14.25	14.12	13.91
3	0.10	0.05	10.13	9.55	9.28	9.12	9.01	8.94	8.89	8.85	8.81	8.79	8.70	8.63	8.53
4	0.05	0.025	12.22	10.65	9.98	9.60	9.36	9.20	9.07	8.98	8.90	8.84	8.66	8.50	8.27
4	0.10	0.05	7.71	6.94	6.59	6.39	6.26	6.16	6.09	6.04	6.00	5.96	5.86	5.77	5.64
5	0.05	0.025	10.01	8.43	7.76	7.39	7.15	6.98	6.85	6.76	6.68	6.62	6.43	6.27	6.03
5	0.10	0.05	6.61	5.79	5.41	5.19	5.05	4.95	4.88	4.82	4.77	4.74	4.62	4.52	4.37
6	0.05	0.025	8.81	7.26	6.60	6.23	5.99	5.82	5.70	5.60	5.52	5.46	5.27	5.11	4.86
6	0.10	0.05	5.99	5.14	4.76	4.53	4.39	4.28	4.21	4.15	4.10	4.06	3.94	3.83	3.68
7	0.05	0.025	8.07	6.54	5.89	5.52	5.29	5.12	4.99	4.90	4.82	4.76	4.57	4.40	4.16
7	0.10	0.05	5.59	4.74	4.35	4.12	3.97	3.87	3.79	3.73	3.68	3.64	3.51	3.40	3.24
8	0.05	0.025	7.57	6.06	5.42	5.05	4.82	4.65	4.53	4.43	4.36	4.30	4.10	3.94	3.68
8	0.10	0.05	5.32	4.46	4.07	3.84	3.69	3.58	3.50	3.44	3.39	3.35	3.22	3.11	2.94
9	0.05	0.025	7.21	5.71	5.08	4.72	4.48	4.32	4.20	4.10	4.03	3.96	3.77	3.60	3.35
9	0.10	0.05	5.12	4.26	3.86	3.63	3.48	3.37	3.29	3.23	3.18	3.14	3.01	2.89	2.72
10	0.05	0.025	6.94	5.46	4.83	4.47	4.24	4.07	3.95	3.85	3.78	3.72	3.52	3.35	3.09
10	0.10	0.05	4.96	4.10	3.71	3.48	3.33	3.22	3.14	3.07	3.02	2.98	2.85	2.73	2.55
15	0.05	0.025	6.20	4.77	4.15	3.80	3.58	3.41	3.29	3.20	3.12	3.06	2.86	2.69	2.41
15	0.10	0.05	4.54	3.68	3.29	3.06	2.90	2.79	2.71	2.64	2.59	2.54	2.40	2.28	2.08
20	0.05	0.025	5.87	4.46	3.86	3.51	3.29	3.13	3.01	2.91	2.84	2.77	2.57	2.40	2.10
20	0.10	0.05	4.35	3.49	3.10	2.87	2.71	2.60	2.51	2.45	2.39	2.35	2.20	2.07	1.86
30	0.05	0.025	5.57	4.18	3.59	3.25	3.03	2.87	2.75	2.65	2.57	2.51	2.31	2.12	1.81
30	0.10	0.05	4.17	3.32	2.92	2.69	2.53	2.42	2.33	2.27	2.21	2.16	2.01	1.88	1.64
50	0.05	0.025	5.34	3.97	3.39	3.05	2.83	2.67	2.55	2.46	2.38	2.32	2.11	1.92	1.57
50	0.10	0.05	4.03	3.18	2.79	2.56	2.40	2.29	2.20	2.13	2.07	2.03	1.87	1.73	1.46
100	0.05	0.025	5.18	3.83	3.25	2.92	2.70	2.54	2.42	2.32	2.24	2.18	1.97	1.77	1.38
100	0.10	0.05	3.94	3.09	2.70	2.46	2.31	2.19	2.10	2.03	1.97	1.93	1.77	1.62	1.31
1000	0.05	0.025	5.04	3.70	3.13	2.80	2.58	2.42	2.30	2.20	2.13	2.06	1.85	1.64	1.16
1000	0.10	0.05	3.85	3.00	2.61	2.38	2.22	2.11	2.02	1.95	1.89	1.84	1.68	1.52	1.13

Derived using Microsoft Excel Version 5.0.

Table A7 Ranks for confidence intervals for the median.

Sample size	Approximate		
	90%CI	95%CI	99%CI
6	1,6	1,6	—
7	1,7	1,7	—
8	2,7	1,8	—
9	2,8	2,8	1,9
10	2,9	2,9	1,10
11	3,9	2,10	1,11
12	3,10	3,10	2,11
13	4,10	3,11	2,12
14	4,11	3,12	2,13
15	4,12	4,12	3,13
16	5,12	4,13	3,14
17	5,13	4,14	3,15
18	6,13	5,14	4,15
19	6,14	5,15	4,16
20	6,15	6,15	4,17
21	7,15	6,16	5,17
22	7,16	6,17	5,18
23	8,16	7,17	5,19
24	8,17	7,18	6,19
25	8,18	8,18	6,20
26	9,18	8,19	6,21
27	9,19	8,20	7,21
28	10,19	9,20	7,22
29	10,20	9,21	8,22
30	11,20	10,21	8,23
31	11,21	10,22	8,24
32	11,22	10,23	9,24
33	12,22	11,23	9,25
34	12,23	11,24	9,26
35	12,23	12,24	10,26
36	13,24	12,25	10,27
37	14,24	13,25	11,27
38	14,25	13,26	11,28
39	14,26	13,27	11,29
40	15,26	14,27	12,29
41	15,27	14,28	12,30
42	16,27	15,28	13,30
43	16,28	15,29	13,31
44	17,28	15,30	13,32
45	17,29	16,30	14,32
46	17,30	16,31	14,33
47	18,30	17,31	15,33
48	18,31	17,32	15,34
49	19,31	18,32	15,35
50	19,32	18,33	16,35

Derived using Microsoft Excel Version 5.0.

Table A8 Wilcoxon signed ranks test.

n'	Two-tailed P-value		
	0.05	0.01	0.001
6	0–21	—	—
7	2–26	—	—
8	3–33	0–36	—
9	5–40	1–44	—
10	8–47	3–52	—
11	10–56	5–61	0–66
12	13–65	7–71	1–77
13	17–74	9–82	2–89
14	21–84	12–93	4–101
15	25–95	15–105	6–114
16	29–107	19–117	9–127
17	34–119	23–130	11–142
18	40–131	27–144	14–157
19	46–144	32–158	18–172
20	52–158	37–173	21–189
21	58–173	42–189	26–205
22	66–187	48–205	30–223
23	73–203	54–222	35–241
24	81–219	61–239	40–260
25	89–236	68–257	45–280

Adapted from Altman, D.G. (1991) *Practical Statistics for Medical Research.* Chapman and Hall, London, with permission.

Table A9(a) Wilcoxon rank sum test for a two-tailed $P = 0.05$.

n_L	\multicolumn{12}{c}{n_s (the number of observations in the smaller sample)}
	4	5	6	7	8	9	10	11	12	13	14	15
4	10–26	16–34	23–43	31–53	40–64	49–77	60–90	72–104	85–119	99–135	114–152	130–170
5	11–29	17–38	24–48	33–58	42–70	52–83	63–97	75–112	89–127	103–144	118–162	134–181
6	12–32	18–42	26–52	34–64	44–76	55–89	66–104	79–119	92–136	107–153	122–172	139–191
7	13–35	20–45	27–57	36–69	46–82	57–96	69–111	82–127	96–144	111–162	127–181	144–201
8	14–38	21–49	29–61	38–74	49–87	60–102	72–118	85–135	100–152	115–171	131–191	149–211
9	14–42	22–53	31–65	40–79	51–93	62–109	75–125	89–142	104–160	119–180	136–200	154–221
10	15–45	23–57	32–70	42–84	53–99	65–115	78–132	92–150	107–169	124–188	141–209	159–231
11	16–48	24–61	34–74	44–89	55–105	68–121	81–139	96–157	111–177	128–197	145–219	164–241
12	17–51	26–64	35–79	46–94	58–110	71–127	84–146	99–165	115–185	132–206	150–228	169–251
13	18–54	27–68	37–83	48–99	60–116	73–134	88–152	103–172	119–193	136–215	155–237	174–261
14	19–57	28–72	38–88	50–104	62–122	76–140	91–159	106–180	123–201	141–223	160–246	179–271
15	20–60	29–76	40–92	52–109	65–127	79–146	94–166	110–187	127–209	145–232	164–256	184–281

Table A9(b) Wilcoxon rank sum test for a two-tailed $P = 0.01$.

n_L	\multicolumn{12}{c}{n_s (the number of observations in the smaller sample)}
	4	5	6	7	8	9	10	11	12	13	14	15
4	—	—	21–45	28–56	37–67	46–80	57–93	68–108	81–123	94–140	109–157	125–175
5	—	15–40	22–50	29–62	38–74	48–87	59–101	71–116	84–132	98–149	112–168	128–187
6	10–34	16–44	23–55	31–67	40–80	50–94	61–109	73–125	87–141	101–159	116–178	132–198
7	10–38	16–49	24–60	32–73	42–86	52–101	64–116	76–133	90–150	104–169	120–188	136–209
8	11–48	17–53	25–65	34–78	43–93	54–108	66–124	79–141	93–159	108–178	123–199	140–220
9	11–45	18–57	26–70	35–84	45–99	56–115	68–132	82–149	96–168	111–188	127–209	144–231
10	12–48	19–61	27–75	37–89	47–105	58–122	71–139	84–158	99–177	115–197	131–219	149–241
11	12–52	20–65	28–80	38–95	49–111	61–128	73–147	87–166	102–186	118–207	135–229	153–252
12	13–55	21–69	30–84	40–100	51–117	63–135	76–154	90–174	105–195	122–216	143–249	162–273
13	13–59	22–73	31–89	41–106	53–123	65–142	79–161	93–182	109–203	125–226	147–259	166–284
14	14–62	22–78	32–94	43–111	54–130	67–149	81–169	96–190	112–212	129–235	151–269	171–294
15	15–65	23–82	33–99	44–117	56–136	69–156	84–176	99–198	115–221	133–244	151–269	171–294

Extracted from *Geigy Scientific Tables*, Vol. 2 (1990), 8th edn, Ciba-Geigy Ltd. with permission.

Table A10 Pearson's correlation coefficient.

Sample size	Two-tailed P-value		
	0.05	0.01	0.001
5	0.878	0.959	0.991
6	0.811	0.917	0.974
7	0.755	0.875	0.951
8	0.707	0.834	0.925
9	0.666	0.798	0.898
10	0.632	0.765	0.872
11	0.602	0.735	0.847
12	0.576	0.708	0.823
13	0.553	0.684	0.801
14	0.532	0.661	0.780
15	0.514	0.641	0.760
16	0.497	0.623	0.742
17	0.482	0.606	0.725
18	0.468	0.590	0.708
19	0.456	0.575	0.693
20	0.444	0.561	0.679
21	0.433	0.549	0.665
22	0.423	0.537	0.652
23	0.413	0.526	0.640
24	0.404	0.515	0.629
25	0.396	0.505	0.618
26	0.388	0.496	0.607
27	0.381	0.487	0.597
28	0.374	0.479	0.588
29	0.367	0.471	0.579
30	0.361	0.463	0.570
35	0.334	0.430	0.532
40	0.312	0.403	0.501
45	0.294	0.380	0.474
50	0.279	0.361	0.451
55	0.266	0.345	0.432
60	0.254	0.330	0.414
70	0.235	0.306	0.385
80	0.220	0.286	0.361
90	0.207	0.270	0.341
100	0.217	0.283	0.357
150	0.160	0.210	0.266

Extracted from *Geigy Scientific Tables*, Vol 2 (1990), 8th edn, Ciba-Geigy Ltd. with permission.

Table A11 Spearman's correlation coefficient.

Sample size	Two tailed P-value		
	0.05	0.01	0.001
5	1.000		
6	0.886	1.000	
7	0.786	0.929	1.000
8	0.738	0.881	0.976
9	0.700	0.833	0.933
10	0.648	0.794	0.903

Adapted from Siegel, S. & Castellan, N.J. (1988) *Nonparametric Statistics for the Behavioural Sciences*, 2nd edn, McGraw-Hill, New York, and used with permission of McGraw-Hill Companies.

Table A12 Random numbers.

3 4 8 1 4	6 8 0 2 0	2 8 9 9 8	5 1 6 8 7	4 0 0 8 8	3 5 4 5 8	2 4 7 0 8	0 1 8 1 5	5 3 7 7 6
9 9 1 0 6	5 0 8 9 9	0 7 3 9 4	9 1 0 7 1	2 2 4 1 1	6 1 6 4 3	6 4 4 3 5	6 2 5 5 2	6 4 3 1 6
4 7 1 8 5	3 1 7 8 2	4 8 8 9 4	6 8 7 9 0	5 1 8 5 2	3 6 9 1 8	0 5 7 3 7	9 0 6 5 3	6 1 1 2 3
8 1 3 5 4	5 7 2 9 6	3 9 3 2 9	5 2 2 6 3	4 3 1 9 4	5 1 6 2 4	4 2 4 2 9	6 1 3 6 7	4 1 2 0 7
8 3 4 6 7	8 5 6 2 2	9 5 7 7 8	0 5 3 4 7	0 0 4 4 5	5 1 3 3 4	2 9 4 4 5	9 9 1 7 6	3 0 0 9 1
2 7 9 2 4	3 4 1 6 7	5 7 0 6 0	5 7 5 3 5	3 2 2 7 8	1 6 9 4 9	0 4 9 6 0	0 4 1 1 6	9 1 4 6 7
5 8 3 1 9	8 8 1 6 4	9 4 1 3 0	0 7 7 4 3	1 6 9 1 7	1 5 6 8 1	9 3 5 7 2	9 9 7 5 3	4 9 1 1 7
4 9 7 3 2	6 6 7 0 2	7 2 4 2 5	9 9 1 1 7	4 9 2 9 8	8 7 2 6 5	1 4 1 9 5	8 3 3 9 1	1 9 7 9 4
6 9 5 9 4	2 6 7 4 9	6 8 7 4 3	3 9 1 3 9	4 4 4 9 5	1 1 9 4 4	1 2 9 7 0	5 6 5 2 3	6 2 4 1 1
3 0 0 7 4	9 7 5 1 7	9 7 4 5 0	5 4 2 5 1	5 1 7 7 7	2 1 0 7 3	0 3 9 0 9	2 6 5 1 9	3 9 5 7 8
8 1 1 4 7	5 7 5 0 8	9 3 4 7 9	8 7 8 2 6	2 8 9 6 5	7 4 4 7 4	9 7 4 6 8	8 0 1 4 9	1 7 8 3 4
7 4 6 8 9	2 8 9 3 3	5 9 8 1 9	9 3 0 5 2	6 1 3 2 5	8 3 1 4 5	4 4 6 8 4	7 2 9 5 8	9 1 8 2 4
1 4 8 0 2	2 5 9 8 2	4 8 0 2 4	1 5 4 6 1	3 7 5 7 0	4 4 6 8 5	4 7 3 8 6	0 9 5 0 4	7 7 8 3 1
6 8 5 0 1	3 4 1 9 4	8 5 3 5 5	3 8 4 1 1	4 6 5 5 9	4 1 6 9 4	9 9 6 7 8	8 8 2 6 8	8 6 6 7 4
4 8 7 3 4	9 2 6 7 1	8 5 2 5 2	8 5 9 8 5	3 4 2 2 8	9 1 2 8 9	5 6 3 3 1	1 4 6 8 3	3 6 4 9 3
8 4 1 0 2	8 1 6 9 9	9 7 3 5 2	5 4 5 0 9	9 3 1 9 6	5 1 2 0 4	4 3 3 5 1	1 1 8 1 8	4 1 1 7 9
2 8 4 3 2	3 2 8 7 3	8 3 8 3 4	0 9 8 6 2	1 2 7 2 0	6 4 5 6 9	4 2 2 1 8	2 6 7 2 6	8 0 8 6 6
9 1 4 5 8	8 2 5 2 4	7 5 5 2 3	0 1 2 7 6	1 9 5 9 1	4 7 4 7 3	9 0 2 5 1	9 9 1 0 3	7 2 9 4 7
4 5 4 3 5	3 0 3 8 9	6 9 7 3 2	8 1 9 6 2	3 0 2 4 3	9 6 1 9 9	3 3 5 4 6	3 9 6 7 2	8 3 7 6 0
2 3 5 5 7	7 8 4 3 7	4 4 9 5 7	9 8 7 2 8	6 5 6 7 4	3 4 7 0 1	8 3 3 9 8	5 4 1 0 2	6 5 8 4 5
3 0 3 9 5	9 1 8 5 0	5 2 0 0 4	0 4 8 4 4	2 8 8 4 8	1 9 7 2 8	9 6 5 7 1	1 3 3 1 7	7 0 8 5 9
6 9 9 9 1	1 2 7 5 5	9 7 9 1 6	5 7 6 3 9	4 3 4 4 5	9 0 4 6 3	8 5 5 5 6	3 5 4 6 9	1 9 7 4 9
3 2 9 8 0	4 3 6 0 8	2 0 5 9 2	7 2 5 2 7	6 3 5 8 3	4 6 4 4 3	5 3 9 2 9	8 7 2 1 9	5 5 1 9 8
5 9 7 7 6	3 7 0 3 5	5 3 7 6 5	5 5 1 9 6	6 8 6 5 9	7 1 4 2 9	2 5 2 2 5	9 1 9 4 2	5 1 1 3 2
7 3 7 1 4	7 9 8 6 8	2 3 8 8 0	9 2 2 5 4	7 2 9 8 4	0 7 7 9 2	8 1 3 0 6	2 4 2 7 7	8 2 3 6 6
6 1 5 4 7	1 6 5 7 5	6 8 5 2 0	5 9 8 6 9	6 7 2 9 9	7 3 5 6 5	7 7 3 1 6	9 6 6 8 2	1 8 0 3 1
8 7 7 3 7	0 1 0 5 8	7 6 0 1 2	7 6 2 4 7	7 5 6 1 6	5 1 3 3 5	7 0 3 6 4	7 8 9 4 2	4 0 5 6 4
9 8 6 6 9	0 8 3 3 4	4 0 5 2 0	7 8 3 8 9	5 6 4 9 8	7 4 3 3 6	0 2 4 3 4	4 8 5 9 9	6 7 5 7 9
8 1 5 3 5	4 6 6 9 0	9 2 8 1 4	4 4 4 5 6	2 9 2 2 7	4 8 1 2 2	3 0 5 2 2	1 3 8 5 2	4 8 4 3 6
0 5 9 7 5	4 7 1 1 0	3 2 7 3 3	4 6 9 2 9	9 8 2 6 1	5 2 1 9 3	8 3 2 1 5	5 3 1 9 2	8 3 1 0 9

Derived using Microsoft Excel Version 5.0.

Appendix B: Altman's nomogram for sample size calculations (Topic 33)

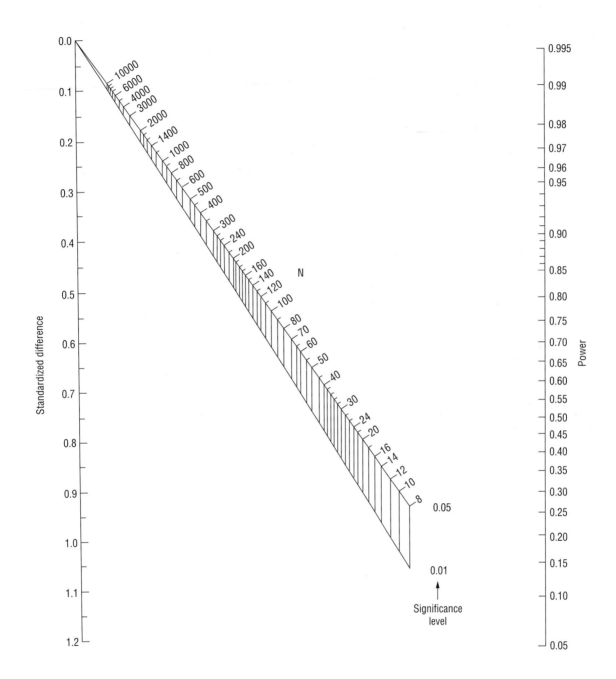

Extracted from: Altman, D.G. (1982) How large a sample? In: *Statistics in Practice* (eds S.M. Gore & D.G. Altman). BMA, London. Copyright BMJ Publishing Group, with permission.

Appendix C: Typical computer output

Analysis of pocket depth data described in Topic 20, generated by SPSS

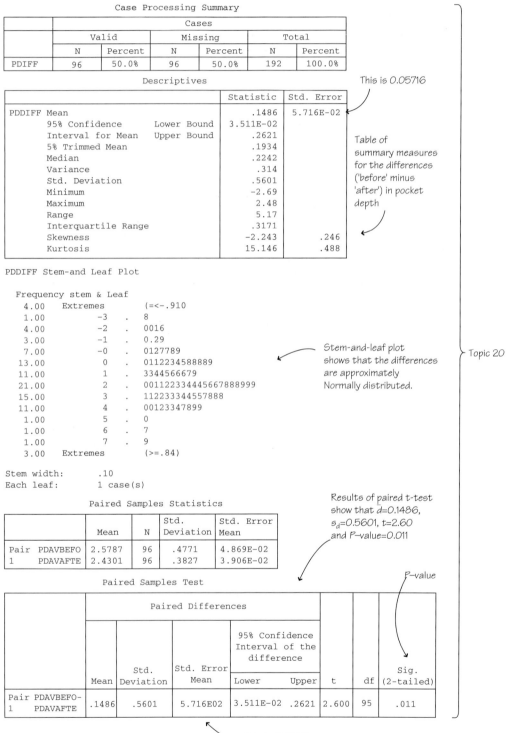

Case Processing Summary

	Cases					
	Valid		Missing		Total	
	N	Percent	N	Percent	N	Percent
PDIFF	96	50.0%	96	50.0%	192	100.0%

Descriptives

			Statistic	Std. Error
PDDIFF	Mean		.1486	5.716E-02
	95% Confidence	Lower Bound	3.511E-02	
	Interval for Mean	Upper Bound	.2621	
	5% Trimmed Mean		.1934	
	Median		.2242	
	Variance		.314	
	Std. Deviation		.5601	
	Minimum		-2.69	
	Maximum		2.48	
	Range		5.17	
	Interquartile Range		.3171	
	Skewness		-2.243	.246
	Kurtosis		15.146	.488

This is 0.05716

Table of summary measures for the differences ('before' minus 'after') in pocket depth

PDDIFF Stem-and Leaf Plot

```
   Frequency  stem & Leaf
       4.00   Extremes        (=<-.910
       1.00      -3  .  8
       4.00      -2  .  0016
       3.00      -1  .  0.29
       7.00      -0  .  0127789
      13.00       0  .  0112234588889
      11.00       1  .  3344566679
      21.00       2  .  001122334445667888999
      15.00       3  .  112233344557888
      11.00       4  .  00123347899
       1.00       5  .  0
       1.00       6  .  7
       1.00       7  .  9
       3.00   Extremes        (>=.84)

   Stem width:       .10
   Each leaf:     1 case(s)
```

Stem-and-leaf plot shows that the differences are approximately Normally distributed.

Paired Samples Statistics

		Mean	N	Std. Deviation	Std. Error Mean
Pair 1	PDAVBEFO	2.5787	96	.4771	4.869E-02
	PDAVAFTE	2.4301	96	.3827	3.906E-02

Results of paired t-test show that d=0.1486, s_d=0.5601, t=2.60 and P-value=0.011

Paired Samples Test

	Paired Differences					t	df	Sig. (2-tailed)
				95% Confidence Interval of the difference				
	Mean	Std. Deviation	Std. Error Mean	Lower	Upper			
Pair 1 PDAVBEFO- PDAVAFTE	.1486	.5601	5.716E02	3.511E-02	.2621	2.600	95	.011

P-value

This is 0.05716

Topic 20

Analysis of platelet data described in Topic 22, generated by SPSS

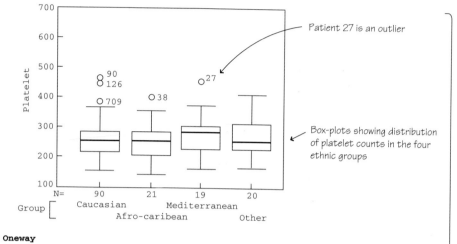

Patient 27 is an outlier

Box-plots showing distribution of platelet counts in the four ethnic groups

Oneway

Platelet

Report

Group	Mean	N	Std. Deviation	Std. Error Of Mean
Caucasian	268.1000	90	77.0784	8.1248
Afro-caribbean	254.2857	21	67.5005	14.7298
Mediterranean	281.0526	19	71.0934	16.3099
Other	273.3000	20	63.4243	14.1821
Total	268.5000	150	73.0451	5.9641

Summary measures for each of the four groups

Platelet   Test of Homogeneity of Variances

Levene Statistic	df1	df2	Sig.
.041	3	146	.989

Results from Levine's test; the P-value of 0.989 indicates that there is no evidence that the variances are different in the four groups

Platelet   Anova

	Sum of Squares	df	Mean Square	F	Sig.
Between Groups	7711.967	3	2570.656	.477	.699
Within Groups	787289.533	146	5392.394		
Total	795001.500	149			

The ANOVA table

P-value

Topic 22

Analysis of FEV1 data described in Topic 21, generated by SAS

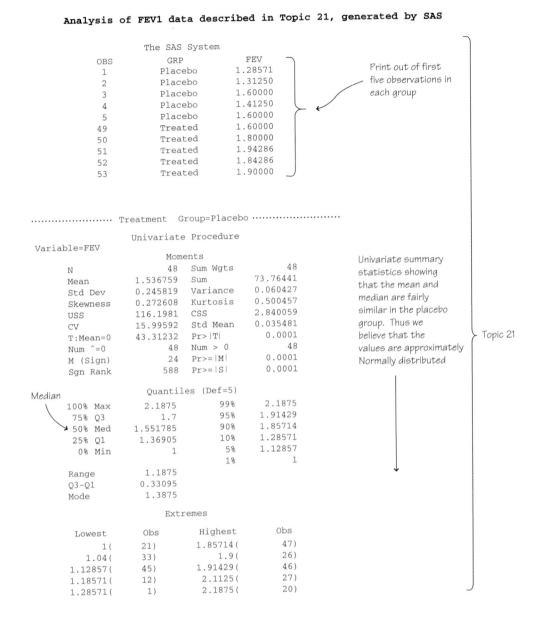

The SAS System

OBS	GRP	FEV
1	Placebo	1.28571
2	Placebo	1.31250
3	Placebo	1.60000
4	Placebo	1.41250
5	Placebo	1.60000
49	Treated	1.60000
50	Treated	1.80000
51	Treated	1.94286
52	Treated	1.84286
53	Treated	1.90000

Print out of first five observations in each group

·············· Treatment Group=Placebo ····················

Univariate Procedure

Variable=FEV

Moments

N	48	Sum Wgts	48
Mean	1.536759	Sum	73.76441
Std Dev	0.245819	Variance	0.060427
Skewness	0.272608	Kurtosis	0.500457
USS	116.1981	CSS	2.840059
CV	15.99592	Std Mean	0.035481
T:Mean=0	43.31232	Pr> |T|	0.0001
Num ^=0	48	Num > 0	48
M (Sign)	24	Pr>= |M|	0.0001
Sgn Rank	588	Pr>= |S|	0.0001

Univariate summary statistics showing that the mean and median are fairly similar in the placebo group. Thus we believe that the values are approximately Normally distributed

Quantiles (Def=5)

Median

100% Max	2.1875	99%	2.1875
75% Q3	1.7	95%	1.91429
50% Med	1.551785	90%	1.85714
25% Q1	1.36905	10%	1.28571
0% Min	1	5%	1.12857
		1%	1
Range	1.1875		
Q3-Q1	0.33095		
Mode	1.3875		

Extremes

Lowest	Obs	Highest	Obs
1(	21)	1.85714(	47)
1.04(	33)	1.9(	26)
1.12857(	45)	1.91429(	46)
1.18571(	12)	2.1125(	27)
1.28571(	1)	2.1875(	20)

Topic 21

continued

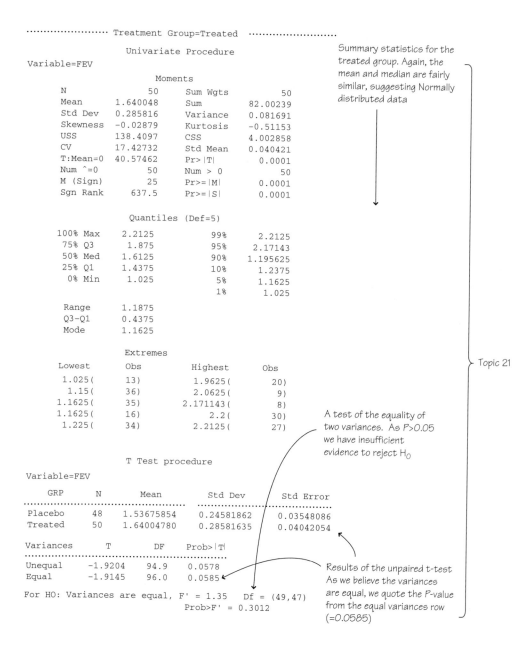

```
················· Treatment Group=Treated  ·····················
                    Univariate Procedure
Variable=FEV
                         Moments
     N                50      Sum Wgts            50
     Mean        1.640048     Sum           82.00239
     Std Dev     0.285816     Variance      0.081691
     Skewness   -0.02879      Kurtosis      -0.51153
     USS          138.4097    CSS           4.002858
     CV          17.42732     Std Mean      0.040421
     T:Mean=0    40.57462     Pr> |T|         0.0001
     Num ^=0           50     Num > 0             50
     M (Sign)          25     Pr>=|M|         0.0001
     Sgn Rank       637.5     Pr>=|S|         0.0001


                      Quantiles (Def=5)

     100% Max     2.2125        99%         2.2125
      75% Q3      1.875         95%         2.17143
      50% Med     1.6125        90%         1.195625
      25% Q1      1.4375        10%         1.2375
       0% Min     1.025          5%         1.1625
                                 1%         1.025

     Range        1.1875
     Q3-Q1        0.4375
     Mode         1.1625

                      Extremes
     Lowest      Obs          Highest        Obs
     1.025(      13)          1.9625(        20)
     1.15 (      36)          2.0625(         9)
     1.1625(     35)          2.171143(       8)
     1.1625(     16)             2.2(        30)
     1.225 (     34)          2.2125(        27)


                    T Test procedure
Variable=FEV
     GRP      N      Mean         Std Dev       Std Error
     ···························  ·················
     Placebo  48   1.53675854   0.24581862    0.03548086
     Treated  50   1.64004780   0.28581635    0.04042054

     Variances      T       DF      Prob>|T|
     ··················  ···········
     Unequal     -1.9204    94.9     0.0578
     Equal       -1.9145    96.0     0.0585

For HO: Variances are equal, F' = 1.35   Df = (49,47)
                              Prob>F' = 0.3012
```

Summary statistics for the treated group. Again, the mean and median are fairly similar, suggesting Normally distributed data

Topic 21

A test of the equality of two variances. As P>0.05 we have insufficient evidence to reject H₀

Results of the unpaired t-test As we believe the variances are equal, we quote the P-value from the equal variances row (=0.0585)

Analysis of anthropometric data described in Topics 26, 28 and 29, generated by SAS

OBS	SBP	Height	Weight	Sex
1	91.00	119.7	20.0	0
2	122.50	124.6	42.5	0
3	109.50	111.3	19.8	0
4	100.50	110.3	18.9	0
5	99.00	112.5	19.0	0
6	103.50	115.1	19.3	0
7	101.00	116.3	19.6	0
8	103.00	111.1	17.1	1
9	106.50	117.2	20.7	1
10	102.50	113.2	22.1	1

Print out of data from first 10 children

Correlation Analysis

4 'VAR' Variables: SBP   Height   Weight   Age

Simple Statistics

Variable	N	Mean	Std Dev	Sum
SBP	100	104.414700	9.430933	10441
Height	100	120.054000	6.439986	12005
Weight	100	22.826000	4.223303	2282.600000
Age	100	6.696900	0.731717	669.690000

Simple Statistics

Variable	Minimum	Maximum
SBP	81.500000	128.850000
Height	107.1000000	136.800000
Weight	15.900000	42.500000
Age	5.130000	8.840000

Summary statistics for each variable

Pearson Correlation Coefficients/Prob> |R| under Ho:Rho=0 /N=100

	SBP	Height	Weight	Age
SBP	1.00000	0.33066	0.51774	0.16373
	0.0	0.0008	0.0001	0.1036
Height	0.33066	1.00000	0.69151	0.64486
	0.0008	0.0	0.0001	0.0001
Weight	0.51774	0.69151	1.00000	0.38935
	0.0001	0.0001	0.0	0.0001
Age	0.16373	0.64486	0.38935	1.00000
	0.1036	0.0001	0.0001	0.0

Pearson's correlation coefficient between SBP and age

Associated P-value

Spearman Correlation Coefficients/Prob> |R| under Ho:Rho=0 /N=100

	SBP	Height	Weight	Age
SBP	1.00000	0.31519	0.45453	0.14778
	0.0	0.0014	0.0001	0.1423
Height	0.31519	1.00000	0.82298	0.61491
	0.0014	0.0	0.0001	0.0001
Weight	0.45453	0.82298	1.00000	0.51260
	0.0001	0.0001	0.0	0.0001
Age	0.14778	0.61491	0.51260	1.00000
	0.1423	0.0001	0.0001	0.0

Spearman's correlation coefficient between height and age

P-value

Topic 26

```
Model:MODEL1
Dependent Variable:SBP
                    Analysis of Variance

Source        DF        Sum of         Mean      F Value    Prob>F
                        Squares        Square
Model          1       962.71441     962.71441    12.030    0.0008       } Anova table
Error         98      7842.59208      80.02645
C Total       99      8805.30649

         Root MSE        8.94575      R-square     0.1093
         Dep Mean      104.41470      Adj R-sq     0.1002
             C.V.        8.56752

                    Parameter Estimates

  Intercept, a

                   Parameter      Standard      T for HO:
Variable    DF     Estimate         Error       Parameter=0

Intercep     1     46.281684     16.78450788      2.757
Height       1      0.484224      0.13960927      3.468

Variable DF        Prob> |T|            Slope, b

Intercep     1      0.0070
Height       1      0.0008
```

Results from simple linear regression of SBP (systolic blood pressure) on height Topic 28

```
Model:MODEL1
Dependent Variable:SBP
                    Analysis of Variance

Source        DF        Sum of         Mean      F Value    Prob>F
                        Squares        Square
Model          3      2804.04514     934.68171    14.952    0.0001
Error         96      6001.26135      62.51314
C Total       99      8805.30649

Root MSE          7.90653          R-square     0.3184
Dep Mean        104.41470          Adj R-sq     0.2972
C.V.              7.57223

                    Parameter Estimates

              Parameter      Standard      T for HO:
Variable    DF   Estimate       Error       Parameter=0

Intercep     1    79.439541    17.11822110      4.641
Height       1    -0.031023     0.17170250     -0.181
Weight       1     1.179495     0.26139400      4.512
Sex          1     4.229540     1.61054848      2.626

Variable    DF   Prob> |T|          Estimated partial
                                    regression
Intercep     1    0.0001            coefficients
Height       1    0.8570
Weight       1    0.0001
Sex          1    0.0101
```

Results from multiple linear regression of SBP on height, weight and gender Topic 29

Analysis of HHV-8 data described in Topics 23, 24 and 30, generated by STATA

.List hhv8 gonorrho syphilis hsv2 hiv age in 1/10

	hhv8	gonorrho	syphilis	hsv2	hiv	age
1.	negative	history	0	0	0	28
2.	negative	history	0	0	0	40
3.	negative	history	0	0	0	26
4.	negative	history	0	1	0	42
5.	positive	history	0	0	0	30
6.	negative	nohistory	0	0	0	33
7.	negative	history	0	1	0	27
8.	positive	history	0	0	0	32
9.	negative	history	1	0	0	35
10.	positive	history	0	0	0	35

Print out of data from first 10 men

. Tabulate gonorrho hhv8, chi row col

Contingency table

gonorrhoe	hhv8 negative	positive	Total
History	192	36	228
Row %	84.21	15.79	100.00
Column %	86.88	72.00	84.13
No history	29	14	43
	67.44	32.56	100.00
	13.12	28.00	15.87
Total	221	50	271
	81.55	18.45	100.00
	100.00	100.00	100.00

Row marginal total → 228
Observed frequency → 14
Column marginal total → 50
Overall total → 271

Topic 24

Pearson chi2(1) = 6.7609 Pr = 0.009

. Logit hhv8 gonorrho syphilis hsv2 hiv age, or tab

```
Interation 0:  Log Likelihood = -122.86506
Interation 1:  Log Likelihood = -111.87072
Interation 2:  Log Likelihood = -110.58712
Interation 3:  Log Likelihood = -110.56596
Interation 4:  Log Likelihood = -110.56595
```

Logit Estimates

Logit Likelihood = -110.56595

Number of obs = 260
chi2 (5) = 24.60
Prob > chi2 = 0.0002
Pseudo R2 = 0.1001

Chi-square for covariates and its P-value

hhv8	Coef.	Std. Err.	z	P>|z|	[95% Conf. Interval]
gonorrho	.5093263	.4363219	1.167	0.243	-.345849 1.364502
syphilis	1.192442	.7110707	1.677	0.094	-.201231 2.586115
hsv2	.7910041	.3871114	2.043	0.041	.0322798 1.549728
hiv	1.635669	.6028147	2.713	0.007	.4541736 2.817164
age	.0061609	.0204152	0.302	0.763	-.0338521 .046174
constant	-2.224164	.6511603	-3.416	0.001	-3.500415 -.9479135

P-value

hhv8	Odds Ratio	Std. Err.	z	P>|z|	[95% Conf. Interval]
gonorrho	1.66417	.7261137	1.167	0.243	.7076193 3.913772
syphilis	3.295118	2.343062	1.677	0.094	.8177235 13.27808
hsv2	2.20561	.8538167	2.043	0.041	1.032806 4.710191
hiv	5.132889	3.094181	2.713	0.007	1.574871 16.72934
age	1.00618	.0205413	0.302	0.763	.9667145 1.047257

CI for odds ratio

Results from multiple logistic regression Topic 30

Comparison of outcomes and probabilites

Outcome	Pr < .5	Pr > = .5	Total
Failure	208	5	213
Success	38	9	47
Total	246	14	260

Predicted outcome
<0.5 = 0 (No)
≥0.5 = 1 (Yes)

Observed outcome Failure = 0 (No)
Success = 1 (Yes)

Classification table

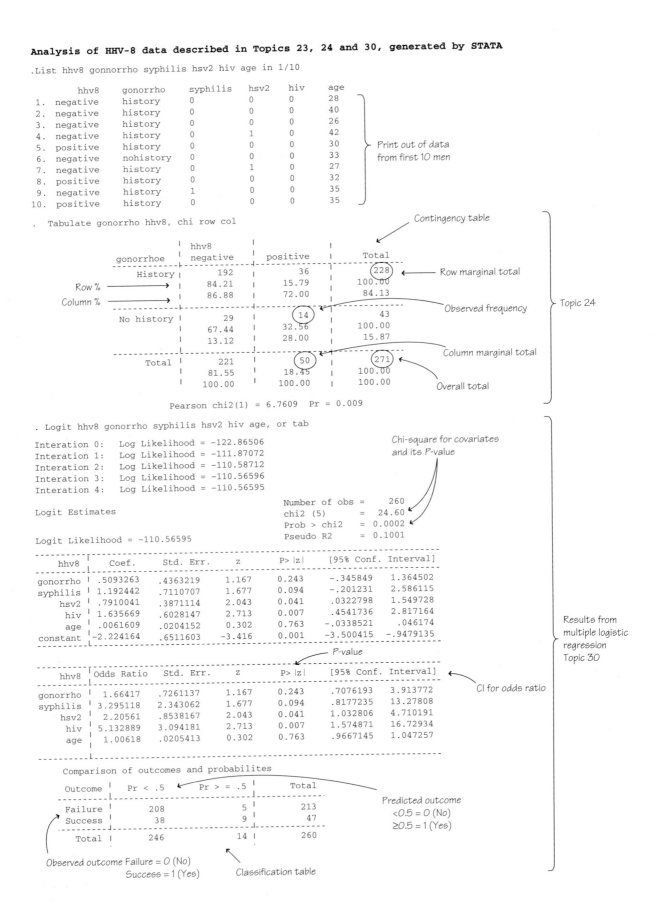

Appendix D: Glossary of terms

2 × 2 table: A contingency table of frequencies with two rows and two columns

Accuracy: Refers to the way in which an observed value of a quantity agrees with the true value

All subsets model selection: See model selection

Allocation bias: A systematic distortion of the data resulting from the way in which individuals are assigned to treatment groups

Alternative hypothesis: The hypothesis about the effect of interest that disagrees with the null hypothesis and is true if the null hypothesis is false

Altman's nomogram: A diagram that relates the sample size of a statistical test to the power, significance level and the standardized difference

Analysis of covariance: A special form of analysis of variance that compares values of a dependent variable between groups of individuals after adjusting for the effect of one or more explanatory variables

Analysis of variance (ANOVA): A general term for analyses that compare means of groups of observations by splitting the total variance of a variable into its component parts, each attributed to a particular factor

ANOVA: See analysis of variance

Arithmetic mean: A measure of location obtained by dividing the sum of the observations by the number of observations. Often called the mean

ASCII or text file format: Data are available on the computer as rows of text

Autocorrelation coefficient of lag k: The correlation coefficient between observations in a time series that are k time units apart

Automatic model selection: A method of selecting variables to be included in a mathematical model, e.g. forwards, backwards, stepwise, all subsets

Average: A general term for a measure of location

Backwards selection: See model selection

Bar or column chart: A diagram that illustrates the distribution of a categorical or discrete variable by showing a separate horizontal or vertical bar for each 'category', its length being proportional to the (relative) frequency in that 'category'

Bartlett's test: Used to compare variances

Bayes theorem: The posterior probability of an event/hypothesis is proportional to the product of its prior probability and the likelihood

Bayesian approach to inference: Uses not only current information (e.g. from a trial) but also an individual's previous belief (often subjective) about a hypothesis to evaluate the posterior belief in the hypothesis

Bias: A systematic difference between the results obtained from a study and the true state of affairs

Bimodal distribution: Data whose distribution has two 'peaks'

Binary variable: A categorical variable with two categories. Also called a dichotomous variable

Binomial distribution: A discrete probability distribution of a binary random variable; useful for inferences about proportions

Blinding: When the patients, clinicians and the assessors of response to treatment in a clinical trial are unaware of the treatment allocation (double-blind), or when the patient is aware of the treatment received but the assessor of response is not (single blind)

Block: A homogeneous group of experimental units that share similar characteristics. Also called a stratum

Bonferroni correction (adjustment): A *post hoc* adjustment to the *P*-value to take account of the number of tests performed in multiple hypothesis testing situations

Box (box-and-whisker) plot: A diagram illustrating the distribution of a variable; it indicates the median, upper and lower quartiles, and, often, the maximum and minimum values

British Standards Institution repeatability coefficient: The maximum difference that is likely to occur between two repeated measurements

Carry-over effect: The residual effect of the previous treatment in a cross-over trial

Case: An individual with the disease under investigation in a case–control study

Case–control study: Groups of individuals with the disease (the cases) and without the disease (the controls) are identified, and exposures to risk factors in these groups are compared

Categorical (qualitative) variable: Each individual belongs to one of a number of distinct categories of the variable

Cell of a contingency table: The designation of a particular row and a particular column of the table

Censored data: Occur in survival analysis because there is incomplete information on outcome. See right- and left-censored data

Chi-squared (χ^2) distribution: A right skewed continuous distribution characterized by its degrees of freedom; useful for analysing categorical data

Chi-squared test: Used on frequency data. It tests the null hypothesis that there is no association between the factors that define a contingency table. Also used to test differences in proportions

CI: See confidence interval

Clinical heterogeneity: Exists when the trials included in a meta-analysis have differences in the patient population, definition of variables, etc., which create problems of non-compatibility

Clinical trial: Any form of planned experiment on humans that is used to evaluate a new treatment on a clinical outcome

Cluster randomization: Groups of individuals, rather than separate individuals, are randomly (by chance) allocated to treatments

Cochrane Collaboration: An international network of clinicians, methodologists and consumers who continuously update systematic reviews and make them available to others

Coefficient of variation: The standard deviation divided by the mean (often expressed as a percentage)

Cohen's kappa (κ): A measure of agreement between two sets of categorical measurements on the same individuals. If $\kappa = 1$ there is perfect agreement; if $\kappa = 0$, there is no better than chance agreement

Cohort study: A group of individuals, all without the outcome of interest (e.g. disease), is followed (usually prospectively) to study the effect on future outcomes of exposure to a risk factor

Collinearity: Pairs of explanatory variables in a regression analysis are very highly correlated, i.e. with correlation coefficients very close to ±1

Complete randomized design: Experimental units assigned randomly to treatment groups

Conditional probability: The probability of an event, *given* that another event has occurred

Confidence interval (CI) for a parameter: The range of values within which we are (usually) 95% confident that the true population parameter lies. Strictly, after repeated sampling, 95% of the estimates of the parameter lie in the interval

Confidence limits: The upper and lower values of a confidence interval

Confounding: When one or more explanatory variables are related to the outcome and each other so that it is difficult to assess the independent effect of each one on the outcome variable

Contingency table: A (usually) two-way table in which the entries are frequencies

Continuity correction: A correction applied to a test statistic to adjust for the approximation of a discrete distribution by a continuous distribution

Continuous probability distribution: The random variable defining the distribution is continuous

Continuous variable: A numerical variable in which there is no limitation on the values that the variable can take other than that restricted by the degree of accuracy of the measuring technique

Control: An individual without the disease under investigation in a case–control study, or not receiving the new treatment in a clinical trial

Control group: A term used in comparative studies, e.g. clinical trials, to denote a comparison group. See also positive and negative controls

Convenience sample: A group of individuals believed to be representative of the population from which it is selected, but chosen because it is close at hand rather than being randomly selected

Correlation coefficient (Pearson's): A quantitative measure, ranging between −1 and +1, of the extent to which points in a scatter diagram conform to a straight line. See also Spearman's rank correlation coefficient

Correlogram: A two-way plot of the autocorrelation coefficient of lag k against k

Covariate: See independent variable

Cox proportional hazard's regression model: See proportional hazard's regression model

Cross-over design: Each individual receives more than one treatment under investigation, one after the other in random order

Cross-sectional studies: Those that are carried out at a single point in time

Cumulative frequency: The number of individuals who have values below and including the specified value of a variable

Cyclic variation: The values exhibit a pattern that keeps repeating itself after a fixed period

Data: Observations on one or more variables

Deciles: Those values that divide the ordered observations into 10 equal parts

Degrees of freedom (df) of a statistic: the sample size minus the number of parameters that have to be estimated to calculate the statistic—they indicate the extent to which the observations are 'free' to vary

Dependent variable: A variable (usually denoted by y) that is predicted by the explanatory variable in regression analysis. Also called the response or outcome variable

df: See degrees of freedom

Diagnostic test: Used to aid or make a diagnosis of a particular condition

Dichotomous variable: See binary variable

Discrete probability distribution: The random variable defining the distribution takes discrete values

Discrete variable: A numerical variable that can only take integer values

Discriminant analysis: A method, similar to logistic regression, which can be used to identify factors that are significantly associated with a binary response

Distribution-free tests: See non-parametric tests

Dot plot: A diagram in which each observation on a variable is represented by one dot on a horizontal (or vertical) line

Double-blind: See blinding

Dummy variables: A set of binary variables that are created to facilitate the comparison of the three of more categories of a nominal variable in a regression analysis

Effect of interest: The value of the response variable that reflects the comparison of interest, e.g. the difference in means

Empirical distribution: The observed distribution of a variable

Epidemiological studies: Observational studies that assess the relationship between risk factors and disease

Error variation: See residual variation

Estimate: A quantity obtained from a sample that is used to represent a population parameter

Evidence-based medicine (EBM): The use of current best evidence in making decisions about the care of individual patients

Expected frequency: The frequency that is expected under the null hypothesis

Experimental study: The investigator intervenes in some way to affect the outcome

Experimental unit: The smallest group of individuals who can be regarded as independent for analysis purposes

Explanatory variable: A variable (usually denoted by x) that is used to predict the dependent variable in a regression analysis. Also called the independent or predictor variable or a covariate

Factorial experiments: Allow the simultaneous analysis of a number of factors of interest

Fagan's nomogram: A diagram relating the pre-test probability of a diagnostic test result to the likelihood and the post-test probability. It is usually used to convert the former into the latter

False negative: An individual who has the disease but is diagnosed as disease-free

False positive: An individual who is free of the disease but is diagnosed as having the disease

F-distribution: A right skewed continuous distribution characterized by the degrees of freedom of the numerator and denominator of the ratio that defines it; useful for comparing two variances, and more than two means using the analysis of variance

Fisher's exact test: A test that evaluates exact probabilities (i.e. does not rely on approximations to the Chi-squared distribution) in a contingency table (usually a 2×2 table), used when the expected frequencies are small

Fitted value: The predicted value of the response variable in a regression analysis corresponding to the particular value(s) of the explanatory variable(s)

Fixed-effect model: Used in a meta-analysis when there is no evidence of statistical heterogeneity

Forest plot: A diagram used in a meta-analysis showing the estimated effect in each trial and their average (with confidence intervals)

Forwards selection: See model selection

Free format data: Each variable in the computer file is separated from the next by some delimiter, often a space or comma

Frequency: The number of times an event occurs

Frequency distribution: Shows the frequency of occurrence of each possible observation, class of observations, or category, as appropriate

Frequentist probability: Proportion of times an event would occur if we were to repeat the experiment a large number of times

F-test: See variance ratio test

Gaussian distribution: See Normal distribution

Geometric mean: A measure of location for data whose distribution is skewed to the right; it is the antilog of the arithmetic mean of the log data

Gold-standard test: Provides a definitive diagnosis of a particular condition

Goodness-of-fit: A measure of the extent to which the values obtained from a model agree with the observed data

Harmonic analysis: A time series that is represented by the sum of the sine and cosine terms of pre-defined period and amplitude

Hazard: The instantaneous risk of reaching the endpoint in survival analysis

Hazard ratio: See relative hazard

Healthy entrant effect: By choosing disease-free individuals to participate in a study, the response of interest (typically, mortality) is lower at the start of the study than would be expected in the general population

Heterogeneity of variance: Unequal variances

Histogram: A diagram that illustrates the (relative) frequency distribution of a continuous variable by using connected bars. The bar's area is proportional to the (relative) frequency in the range specified by the boundaries of the bar

Historical controls: Individuals who are not assigned to a treatment group at the start of the study, but who received treatment some time in the past, and are used as a comparison group

Homoscedasticity: Equal variances; also described as homogeneity of variance

Hypothesis test: The process of using a sample to assess how much evidence there is against a null hypothesis about the population. Also called a significance test

Incidence: The number of individuals who contract the disease in a particular time period, usually expressed as a proportion of those who are susceptible at the start or mid-point of the period

Incident cases: Patients who have just been diagnosed

Independent samples: Each unit in every sample is represented only once, and is unrelated to the units in the other samples

Independent variable: See explanatory variable

Inference: The process of drawing conclusions about the population using sample data

Influential point: A data value that has the effect of substantially altering the estimates of regression coefficients when it is included in the analysis

Intention-to-treat analysis: All patients in the clinical trial are analysed in the groups to which they were originally assigned

Interaction: This exists between two factors when the difference between the levels of one factor is different for two or more levels of the second factor

Intercept: The value of the dependent variable in a regression equation when the value(s) of the explanatory variable(s) is (are) zero

Interdecile range: The difference between the 10th and 90th percentiles; it contains the central 80% of the ordered observations

Interim analyses: Pre-planned analyses at intermediate stages of a study

Interpolate: Estimate the required value that lies between two known values

Interquartile range: The difference between the 25th and 75th percentiles; it contains the central 50% of the ordered observations

Interval estimate: A range of values within which we believe the population parameter lies.

Jackknifing: A method of estimating parameters in a model; each of n individuals is successively removed from the sample, the parameters are estimated from the remaining $n - 1$ individuals, and finally these estimates are averaged

Kaplan–Meier plot: A survival curve in which the survival probability is plotted against the time from baseline. It is used when exact times to reach the endpoint are known

Kolmogorov–Smirnov test: Determines whether data are Normally distributed

Kruskal–Wallis test: A non-parametric alternative to the one-way ANOVA; used to compare the distributions of more than two independent groups of observations

Left-censored data: Come from patients in whom follow-up did not begin until after the baseline date

Lehr's formulae: Can be used to calculate the optimal sample sizes required for some hypothesis tests when the power is specified as 80% or 90% and the significance level as 0.05

Level: A particular category of a qualitative variable or factor

Levene's test: Tests the null hypothesis that two or more variances are equal

Lifetable approach to survival analysis: A way of determining survival probabilities when the time to reach the end-point is only known to within a particular time interval

Likelihood: Of a hypothesis describes the plausibility of an observed result (e.g. from a test) if the hypothesis is true (e.g. disease is present)

Likelihood ratio (LR): A ratio of two likelihoods; for diagnostic tests, the LR is the ratio of the chances of getting a particular test result in those having and not having the disease

Limits of agreement: In an assessment of repeatability, it is the range of values between which we expect 95% of the differences between repeated measurements in the population to lie

Linear regression line: A straight line drawn on a scatter diagram that is defined by an algebraic expression linking two variables

Linear relationship: Implies a straight line relationship between two variables

Logistic regression: The regression relationship between a binary outcome variable and a number of explanatory variables

Logistic regression coefficient: The partial regression coefficient in a logistic regression

Logit (logistic) transformation: A transformation applied to a proportion or probability, p, such that $\mathrm{logit}(p) = \ln\{p/(1 - p)\}$

Lognormal distribution: A right skewed probability distribution of a random variable whose logarithm follows the Normal distribution

Log-rank test: A non-parametric approach to comparing two survival curves

Longitudinal studies: Follow individuals over a period of time

Main outcome variable: That which relates to the major objective of the study

Mann–Whitney U test: See Wilcoxon rank sum test

Marginal total in a contingency table: The sum of the frequencies in a given row (or column) of the table

Matching: A process of selecting individuals who are similar with respect to variables that may influence the response of interest

McNemar's test: Compares proportions in two related groups using a Chi-squared test statistic

Mean: See arithmetic mean

Median: A measure of location that is the middle value of the ordered observations

Meta-analysis (overview): A quantitative systematic review that combines the results of relevant studies to produce, and investigate, an estimate of the overall effect of interest

Method of least squares: A method of estimating the parameters in a regression analysis, based on minimizing the sum of the squared residuals

Mode: The value of a single variable that occurs most frequently in a data set

Model: Describes, in algebraic terms, the relationship between two or more variables

Model Chi-square (Chi-square for covariates): The test statistic, with a χ^2 distribution, which tests the null hypothesis that all the partial regression coefficients in the model are zero

Multi-level modelling: Hierarchical extension, accounting for complex structures in the data, of regression analysis

Multiple linear regression: A linear regression model in which there is a single dependent variable and two or more explanatory variables

Mutually exclusive categories: Each individual can belong to only one category

Negative controls: Those patients in a randomized controlled trial (RCT) who do not receive active treatment

Negative predictive value: The proportion of individuals with a negative test result who do not have the disease

Nominal variable: A categorical variable whose categories have no natural ordering

Non-parametric tests: Hypothesis tests that do not make assumptions about the distribution of the data. Sometimes called distribution-free tests or rank methods

Normal (Gaussian) distribution: A continuous probability distribution that is bell-shaped and symmetrical; its parameters are the mean and variance

Normal plot: A diagram for assessing, visually, the Normality of data; a straight line on the Normal plot implies Normality

Normal range: See reference interval

Null hypothesis, H_0: The statement that assumes no effect in the population

Number of patients needed to treat (NNT): The number of patients we need to treat with the experimental rather than the control treatment to prevent one of them developing the 'bad' outcome

Numerical (quantitative) variable: A variable that takes either discrete or continuous values

Observational study: The investigator does nothing to affect the outcome

Odds: The ratio of the probabilities of two complimentary events, typically the probability of having a disease divided by the probability of not having the disease

Odds ratio: The ratio of two odds (e.g. the odds of disease in individuals exposed and unexposed to a factor). Often taken as an estimate of the relative risk in a case–control study

One-sample *t*-test: Investigates whether the mean of a variable differs from some hypothesized value

One-tailed test: The alternative hypothesis specifies the direction of the effect of interest

One-way analysis of variance: A particular form of ANOVA used to compare the means of more than two independent groups of observations

On-treatment analysis: Patients in a clinical trial are only included in the analysis if they complete a full course of the treatment to which they were randomly assigned

Ordinal variable: A categorical variable whose categories are ordered in some way

Outlier: An observation that is distinct from the main body of the data, and is incompatible with the rest of the data

Overfitted models: Those that contain too many variables, i.e. more than 1/10th of the number of individuals

Overview: See meta-analysis

Paired observations: Relate to responses from matched individuals or the same individual in two different circumstances

Paired *t*-test: Tests the null hypothesis that the mean of a set of differences of paired observations is equal to zero

Parallel trial: Each patient receives only one treatment

Parameter: A summary measure (e.g. the mean, proportion) that characterizes a probability distribution. Its value relates to the population

Parametric test: Hypothesis test that makes certain distributional assumptions about the data

Partial regression coefficients: The parameters, other than the intercept, which describe a multiple linear regression equation

Pearson's correlation coefficient: See correlation coefficient

Percentage point: The percentile of a distribution; it indicates the proportion of the distribution that lies to its right (i.e. in the right hand tail), to its left (i.e. in the left-hand tail), or in both the right- and left-hand tails

Percentiles: Those values that divide the ordered observations into 100 equal parts

Periodogram: A graphical display used in harmonic analysis, part of time series analysis

Pie chart: A diagram showing the frequency distribution of a categorical or discrete variable. A circular 'pie' is split into sections, one for each 'category'; the area of each section is proportional to the frequency in that category

Placebo: An inert 'treatment' used in a clinical trial that is identical in appearance to the active treatment. It removes the effect of receiving treatment from the therapeutic comparison

Point estimate: A single value, obtained from a sample, which estimates a population parameter

Point prevalence: The number of individuals with a disease (or percentage of those susceptible) at a particular point in time

Poisson distribution: A discrete probability distribution of a random variable representing the number of events occurring randomly and independently at a fixed average rate

Polynomial regression: A non-linear (e.g. quadratic, cubic, quartic) relationship between a dependent variable and an explanatory variable

Population: The entire group of individuals in whom we are interested

Positive controls: Those patients in a RCT who receive some form of active treatment as a basis of comparison for the novel treatment

Positive predictive value: The proportion of individuals with a positive diagnostic test result who have the disease

Posterior probability: An individual's belief, based on prior belief and new information (e.g. a test result), that an event will occur

***Post-hoc* comparison adjustments:** Are made to adjust the *P*-values when multiple comparisons are performed, e.g. Bonferroni

Post-test probability: The posterior probability, determined from previous information and the diagnostic test result, that an individual has a disease

Power: The probability of rejecting the null hypothesis when it is false

Precision: A measure of sampling error. Refers to how well repeated observations agree with one another

Predictor variable: See independent variable

Pre-test probability: The prior probability, evaluated before a diagnostic test result is available, that an individual has a disease

Prevalence: The number (proportion) of individuals with a disease at a given point in time (point prevalence) or within a defined interval (period prevalence)

Prevalent cases: Patients who were diagnosed at some previous time

Primary endpoint: The outcome that most accurately reflects the benefit of a new therapy in a clinical trial

Prior probability: An individual's belief, based on subjective views and/or retrospective observations, that an event will occur

Probability: Measures the chance of an event occurring. It lies between 0 and 1. See also conditional, prior and posterior probability

Probability density function: The equation that defines a probability distribution

Probability distribution: A theoretical distribution that is described by a mathematical model. It shows the probabilities of all possible values of a random variable

Prognostic index: Assesses the likelihood that an individual has a disease. Also called a risk score

Proportion: The ratio of the number of events of interest to the total number of events

Proportional hazards regression model (Cox): Used in survival analysis to study the simultaneous effect of a number of explanatory variables on survival

Prospective study: Individuals are followed forward from some point in time

Protocol: A full written description of all aspects of a clinical trial

Protocol deviations: The patients who enter a clinical trial but do not fulfill the protocol criteria

Publication bias: A tendency for journals to publish only papers that contain statistically significant results

P-value: The probability of obtaining our results, or something more extreme, if the null hypothesis is true

Qualitative variable: See categorical variable

Quantitative variable: See numerical variable

Quartiles: Those values that divide the ordered observations into four equal parts

Quota sampling: Non-random sampling in which the investigator chooses sample members to fulfil a specified 'quota'

R^2: The proportion of the total variation in the dependent variable in a regression analysis that is explained by the model. It is a subjective measure of goodness-of-fit

Random sampling: Every possible sample of a given size in the population has an equal probability of being chosen

Random series: A time series in which there is no autocorrelation

Random variable: A quantity that can take any one of a set of mutually exclusive values with a given probability

Random variation: Variability that cannot be attributed to any explained sources

Random-effects model: Used in a meta-analysis when there is evidence of statistical heterogeneity

Randomized controlled trial (RCT): A comparative clinical trial in which there is random allocation of patients to treatments

Randomization: Patients are allocated to treatment groups in a random (based on chance) manner. May be *stratified* (controlling for the effect of important factors) or *blocked* (ensuring approximately equally sized treatment groups)

Range: The difference between the smallest and largest observations

Rank correlation coefficient: See Spearman's rank correlation coefficient

Rank methods: See non-parametric tests

RCT: See randomized controlled trial

Recall bias: A systematic distortion of the data resulting from the way in which individuals remember past events

Receiver operating characteristic (ROC) curve: A two-way plot of the sensitivity against one minus the specificity for different cut-off values for a continuous variable in a diagnostic test; used to select the optimal cut-off value or to compare tests

Reference interval: The range of values (usually the central 95%) of a variable that are typically seen in healthy individuals. Also called the normal or reference range

Regression coefficients: The parameters (i.e. the slope and intercept in simple regression) that describe a regression equation

Regression to the mean: A phenomenon whereby a subset of extreme results is followed by results that are less extreme on average e.g. tall fathers having shorter (but still tall) sons

Relative frequency: The frequency expressed as a percentage or proportion of the total frequency

Relative hazard: The ratio of two hazards, interpreted in a similar way to the relative risk. Also called the hazard ratio

Relative risk (RR): The ratio of two risks, usually the risk of a disease in a group of individuals exposed to some factor, divided by the risk in unexposed individuals

Repeatability: The extent to which repeated measurements by the same observer in identical conditions agree

Repeated measures: The variable of interest is measured on the same individual in more than one set of circumstances (e.g. on different occasions)

Repeated measures ANOVA: A special form of analysis of variance used when a numerical variable is measured in each member of a group of individuals on a number of different occasions

Replication: The individual has more than one measurement of the variable on a given occasion

Reproducibility: The extent to which the same results can be obtained in different circumstances, e.g. by two methods of measurement, or by two observers

Residual: The difference between the observed and fitted values of the dependent variable in a regression analysis

Residual variation: The variance of a variable that remains after the variability attributable to factors of interest has been removed. It is the variance unexplained by the model, and is the residual mean square in an ANOVA table. Also called the error or unexplained variation

Response variable: See dependent variable

Retrospective studies: Individuals are selected, and factors that have occurred in their past are studied

Right-censored data: Come from patients who were known not to have reached the endpoint of interest when they were last under follow-up

Risk of disease: The probability of developing the disease in the stated time period

Risk score: See prognostic index

Risk factor: A determinant that affects the incidence of a particular outcome, e.g. a disease

Robust: A test is robust to violations of its assumptions if its P-value and the power are not appreciably affected by the violations

RR: See relative risk

Sample: A subgroup of the population

Sampling distribution of the mean: The distribution of the sample means obtained after taking repeated samples of a fixed size from the population

Sampling distribution of the proportion: The distribution of the sample proportions obtained after taking repeated samples of a fixed size from the population

Sampling error: The differences, attributed to taking only a sample of values, between what is observed in the sample and what is present in the population

Sampling frame: A list of all the individuals in the population

Saturated model: One in which the number of variables equals or is greater than the number of individuals

Scatter diagram: The two-dimensional plot of one variable against another, with each pair of observations marked by a point

SD: See standard deviation

Seasonal variation: The values of the variable of interest vary systematically according to the time of the year

Secondary endpoints: The outcomes in a clinical trial that are not of primary importance

Selection bias: A systematic distortion of the data resulting from the way in which individuals are included in a sample

SEM: See standard error of mean

Sensitivity: The proportion of individuals with the disease who are correctly diagnosed by the test

Serial correlation: The correlation between the observations in a time series and those observations lagging behind (or leading) by a fixed time interval

Shapiro–Wilk test: Determines whether data are Normally distributed

Sign test: A non-parametric test that investigates whether differences tend to be positive (or negative); whether observations tend to be greater (or less) than the median; whether the proportion of observations with a characteristic is greater (or less) than one half

Significance level: The probability, chosen at the outset of an investigation, which will lead us to reject the null hypothesis if our *P*-value lies below it. It is often chosen as 0.05

Significance test: See hypothesis test

Simple linear regression: The straight line relationship between a single dependent variable and a single explanatory variable

Single-blind: See blinding

Skewed distribution: The distribution of the data is asymmetrical; it has a long tail to the right with a few high values (*positively* skewed) or a long tail to the left with a few low values (*negatively* skewed)

Slope: The gradient of the regression line, showing the average change in the dependent variable for a unit change in the explanatory variable

SND: See Standardized Normal Deviate

Spearman's rank correlation coefficient: The non-parametric alternative to the Pearson correlation coefficient; it provides a measure of association between two variables

Specificity: The proportion of individuals without the disease who are correctly identified by a diagnostic test

Standard deviation (SD): A measure of spread equal to the square root of the variance

Standard error of the mean (SEM): A measure of precision of the sample mean. It is the standard deviation of the sampling distribution of the mean

Standard error of the proportion: A measure of precision of the sample proportion. It is the standard deviation of the sampling distribution of the proportion

Standard Normal distribution: A particular Normal distribution with a mean of zero and a variance of one

Standardized difference: A ratio, used in Altman's nomogram and Lehr's formulae, which expresses the clinically important treatment difference as a multiple of the standard deviation

Standardized Normal Deviate (SND): A random variable whose distribution is Normal with zero mean and unit variance

Stationary time series: A time series for which the mean and variance are constant over time

Statistic: The sample estimate of a population parameter

Statistical heterogeneity: Is present in a meta-analysis when there is considerable variation between the separate estimates of the effect of interest

Statistically significant: The result of a hypothesis test is statistically significant at a particular level (say 1%) if we have sufficient evidence to reject the null hypothesis at that level (i.e. when $P < 0.01$)

Statistics: Encompasses the methods of collecting, summarizing, analysing and drawing conclusions from data

Stem-and-leaf plot: A mixture of a diagram and a table used to illustrate the distribution of data. It is similar to a histogram, and is effectively the data values displayed in increasing order of size

Stepwise selection: See model selection

Stratum: A subgroup of individuals; usually, the individuals within a stratum share similar characteristics. Sometimes called a block

Student's *t*-distribution: See *t*-distribution

Subjective probability: Personal degree of belief that an event will occur

Survival analysis: Examines the time taken for an individual to reach an endpoint of interest (e.g. death) when some data are censored

Symmetrical distribution: The data are centred around some midpoint, and the shape of the distribution to the left of the midpoint is a mirror image of that to the right of it

Systematic allocation: Patients in a clinical trial are allocated treatments in a systematized, non-random, manner

Systematic review: A formalized and stringent approach to combining the results from all relevant studies of similar investigations of the same health condition

Systematic sampling: The sample is selected from the population using some systematic method rather than that based on chance

***t*-distribution:** Also called Student's *t*-distribution. A continuous distribution whose shape is similar to the Normal distribution and that is characterized by its degrees of freedom. It is particularly useful for inferences about the mean

Test statistic: A quantity, derived from sample data, used to test a hypothesis; its value is compared with a known probability distribution to obtain a *P*-value

Time series: Values of a variable observed either on an individual or a group of individuals at many successive points in time

Training sample: The first subsample used to generate the model (e.g. in logistic regression or discriminant analysis). The results are authenticated by a second (validation) sample

Transformed data: Obtained by taking the same mathematical transformation (e.g. log) of each observation

Treatment effect: The effect of interest (e.g. the difference between means or the relative risk) that affords treatment comparisons

Trend: Values of the variable show a tendency to increase or decrease progressively over time

Two-sample *t*-test: See unpaired *t*-test

Two-tailed test: The direction of the effect of interest is not specified in the alternative hypothesis

Type I error: Rejection of the null hypothesis when it is true

Type II error: Non-rejection of the null hypothesis when it is false

Unbiased: Free from bias

Unexplained variation: See residual variation

Uniform distribution: Has no 'peaks' because each value is equally likely

Unimodal distribution: Has a single 'peak'

Unpaired (two-sample) *t*-test: Tests the null hypothesis that two means from independent groups are equal

Validation sample: A second subsample, used to authenticate the results from the training sample

Validity: Closeness to the truth

Variable: Any quantity that varies

Variance: A measure of spread equal to the square of the standard deviation

Variance ratio (*F*-) test: Used to compare two variances by comparing their ratio to the *F*-distribution

Wald test statistic: Often used in logistic regression to test the contribution of a partial regression coefficient

Washout period: The interval between the end of one treatment period and the start of the second treatment period in a cross-over trial. It allows the residual effects of the first treatment to dissipate

Weighted kappa: A refinement of Cohen's kappa, measuring agreement, which takes into account the extent to which two sets of paired categorical measurements disagree

Weighted mean: A modification of the arithmetic mean, obtained by attaching weights to each value of the variable in the data set

Wilcoxon rank sum (two-sample) test: A non-parametric test comparing the distributions of two independent groups of observations. It is equivalent to the Mann–Whitney *U* test.

Wilcoxon signed ranks test: A non-parametric test comparing paired observations

Index

Page numbers in *italics* refer to figures and those in **bold** refer to tables, where these are separated from their discussion in the text. The alphabetical arrangement is letter-by-letter.

rank methods *see* non-parametric tests
rates 9
ratios 9
RCT (randomized controlled trial) 34, 96
recall bias 31, 38, 41
receiver operating characteristic (ROC) curve 91, *92*
reciprocal transformation 25
reference interval (range) 18, 21, 90
regression
    Cox 107, 108
    linear *see* linear regression
    logistic 78–9, 126
    to mean 71
    models, survival data 106–7
    multiple 70, 75–7, 125
    polynomial 78
    presenting results in 87–8
    simple 70, 72–4
regression coefficients 70
    linear 70
    logistic 78
    partial 75, 76
regression line 70, 72
    goodness-of-fit 70
    prediction from 73, 74
    slope of 70, 72–3, 74
relative hazards 107
relative risk (RR) 38, 39
    in meta-analysis 98, 100
    odds ratio as estimate of 78
reliability 98
    assessing 90
repeatability 93, 94, 95
    coefficient, British Standards Institution 93, 95
repeated measures 101–3
replication 32
reproducibility 93
residual mean square (variance) 55, 71
residuals 70, 72
    random series of 105
residual variance 55, 71
response variables *see* dependent variables
results
    assessing 96–7
    presenting 87–9
retrospective studies 30, 31
risk 38
    factors 37
    relative *see* relative risk
    scores 80–1
robust analysis 46, 82

sample 8, 26
    convenience 26
    random 26
    representative 26
    statistic 26
    training 81
    validation 81
sample size 32, 35
    calculations 84–6, *119*
    importance 84
    power and 44, *45*, 84
sampling 26–7
    distributions 26–7
    error 26
    frame 26
    quota 26
    systematic 26
    variation 26

saturated models 80
scatter diagram 15, 67, 70, 72
Scheffé's test 55
scores 9
screening 71
SD *see* standard deviation
SE *see* standard error
seasonal variation 104
segmented column (bar) chart 14, *15*
selection bias 31, 38
SEM (standard error of mean) 26–27, 87
sensitivity 90, 92
serial correlation 104, 105
Shapiro-Wilk test 82
significance level 42–3, 44
    in sample size calculation 84
significance testing *see* hypothesis testing
significant result 42
sign test 46–7, 48, 112, **114**
    paired data 49–50
    for a proportion 58–9, 60
single-blind trial 34
single-coded variables 10
skewed data 46
    negatively 14, *15*
    positively 14, *16*
    transformations for 24–5
slope, regression line 70, 72–3, 74
Spearman's rank correlation coefficient 68, 69, 113, **117**, 124
specificity 90, 92
spread of data 18–19, 87
square root transformation 24–5
square transformation 25
standard deviation (SD) 19, 27, 87
    pooled 55, 57
standard error (SE) 87
    of mean (SEM) 26–7, 87
    of proportion 27
    of slope 72–3
    vs standard deviation 27
standardized difference 84
Standardized Normal Deviate (SND) 21
Standard Normal distribution 21, 112, **113**, **114**
stationary time series 104
statistic 20
    sample 26
    test 42
statistical tables 112–18
statistics, definition of 8
stem-and-leaf plot 14, *15*, 120
stepwise selection 80
stratified randomization 34
stratum 32
Student's *t*-distribution *see* *t*-distribution
study design *see* design, study
subjective probability 20
summary measures
    of location 16–17
    for repeated measures 101
    of spread 18–19
survival
    analysis 106–8
    curves (Kaplan–Meier) 106, *107*
    probability 106
symmetrical distribution 14, *16*
systematic allocation 34
systematic reviews 98

tables 87
    statistical 112–18

t-distribution 22, 112, **113**
    for confidence interval estimation 28
test statistic
    explanation of 42
    for a specific test *see* hypothesis testing
text format 10
time series 104–5
training sample 81
transformation, data 24–5
treatment 32
    allocation 34
    comparisons 34
    effect 44
    efficacy 34
trend
    Chi-squared test for 64–5, 66
    over time 104
t-test
    one-sample 46, 47
    paired 49, 50, **85**, 120
    for partial regression coefficients 76
    unpaired (two-sample) 52, 53–4, 85–6, 123
2 × 2 table 61, 62–3
two-sample *t*-test 52, 53–4, 85–6, 123
two-tailed test 42
Type I, II errors 44
typing errors 12

unbiased estimate 26
uniform distribution 14
unimodal distribution 14
unit, experimental 32
unpaired *t*-test *see* two-sample *t*-test

validation sample 81
validity 81
variability 18, 44
    sample size calculation and 84
variables 8
    see also data; *specific types*
variance 18–19
    of discrete distributions 23
    heterogeneity of 82, 98
    homogeneity of 82
    residual 55, 71
    stabilizing transformations 24, 25
    testing for equality of two 56, 82, 83, 123
variance-ratio test *see* *F*-test
variation 32
    between-group 55
    between-subject 19
    coefficient of 19
    cyclic 104, 105
    over time 104
    random 32, 104
    sampling 26
    unexplained (residual) 55, 71
    within-group 55
    within-subject 19

Wald test statistic 78
washout period 32
Weibull model 107
Wilcoxon rank sum (two-sample) test 53, 54, 112, **116**
Wilcoxon signed ranks test 47, 49–50, 51, 112, **115**

z-test 46
z value 47, 48, 112, **113**